D1316105

Sirtfood Diet

3 Books in 1

Complete Guide To Burn Fat Activating Your "Skinny Gene"+ 200 Tasty Recipes Cookbook For Quick and Easy Meals + A Smart 4 Weeks Meal Plan To Jumpstart Your Weight Loss.

Kate Hamilton

Copyright © 2020

COPYRIGHT PROTECTION

All rights reserved. No part of this publication may be reproduced, distributed, or transmitted in any form or by any means, including photocopying, recording, or other electronic or mechanical methods, without the prior written permission of the publisher, except in the case of brief quotations embodied in critical reviews and certain other noncommercial uses permitted by copyright law.

Introduction

The Sirtfood Diet has been created by celebrity nutritionists Aidan Goggins and Glen Matten in 2016. Designed to include certain foods that will enable to trigger body's skinny gene, the diet is intended to help people rapidly shed excess weight without the consequences that are commonly seen in other diets.

Some diets require you to starve yourself, causing loss of muscle along with the fat. Others need you to give up on foods that you enjoy, making them so restrictive that they are difficult for most people to keep up with.

On the other hand, the Sirtfood Diet encourages you to focus on sirtuin-rich foods that can be combined into meals that are delicious and satisfying, both for mind and body, making it very sustainable and effective.

With a mild calorie restriction for a short period of time and the increase in sirtuin-rich foods, your body will let go of the excess fat even with low intensity or no exercise. Matten and Goggins in the tests made prior the release of the diet, proved that the vast majority of people lost significant amount of weight: 7 pounds on average.

But it's not just a matter of weight loss, the Sirtfood Diet evidenced to improve mental health and general wellbeing as well. Overall, there are some pretty compelling reasons to start considering the Sirtfood Diet— if you want to lose weight, gain muscle, and be healthier; this is a great way to be able to do this. It will take diligence and dedication, but if you can make sure that you commit to this process, you, too, can reap these benefits. You can begin to be a healthier individual, inside and out.

Chapter 1.   The Sirtfood Diet Explained

The Sirtfood Diet is very famous due to its scientific benefits and amazing transformations within the body's metabolic capacities. Thousands of people have unlocked incredible and aesthetic physiques by following the Sirtfood Diet.

These results are not coming from myths attached to basic philosophies of dieting; in fact, the Sirtfood Diet has a robust yet growing scientific background. It is important to understand how and why it works, so that you can fully appreciate the value of what you are doing to improve your health and wellbeing.

The Process of Fat Burning

The most significant benefit of the Sirtfood Diet is its incredible impact on losing fat from the body. Fat is made up of fatty acids that combine to make adipocytes. These adipocytes are clusters of fatty acids, and unlike free fatty acids, adipocytes are not mostly present in the blood.

They get accumulated under skin, in muscles, and on different organs. These adipocytes combine to make adipose tissue, which is full fledge foam-shaped cluster of visible yellowish white-color fat in our body.

Adipose tissue is the healthiest fat to burn, but to do so, it must have been broken down into adipocytes first and then into free fatty acids in a process called lipolysis. These steps are not easy as they seem, and burning extra pounds of fats can be a hard nut to crack.

The most challenging step in this cycle is to break adipose tissue into adipocytes and this process is aided by compounds named polyphenols.

Polyphenols Action

Polyphenols are well-known chemical compounds that act on an essential lean gene to activate a fat-burning action inside the human body. To be very specific, sirtfoods are those which contain high levels of chemical compounds called polyphenols. These compounds are present naturally in sirtfoods and even if they are not equally distributed, it's true that every sirtfood contains specific amounts of different types of polyphenols.

Polyphenols are essential precursors in the fat burning cycle of the body called lipolysis. During lipolysis, adipose tissue is broken down to free fatty acids that are moved in our

Of course, as you might now anticipate, sirtuins also affect our WAT and BAT levels. More precisely, sirtuins help convert your WAT into BAT, changing your body and making it easier to burn calories and lose weight. Over time this will produce substantial differences in your body composition, helping to not only make you lose weight, but become lean and fit.

Improving the Energy-Boosting Effect

The quantity of energy the body requires depends on an individual's daily activities, psychological factors such as stress, and metabolic rate. Essential body cells and tissues such as the brain need a constant supply of energy to maintain their functions, and the energy-boosting effect can improve the functionality of these vital tissues and cells.

So, the energy-boosting effect refers to all the activities geared towards ensuring constant energy supply to body organs, tissues, and cells. Following the Sirtfood Diet is surely one of these, as it guarantees an abundance of fruits and vegetables, plant and animal proteins, whole grains, and healthy fats which play a significant role in enhancing the energy-boosting effect for a healthy living routine.

Drinking sufficient water improves the energy-boosting effect too. Water is a significant component in every food consumed. Keeping hydrated is essential for body health. Water requirement in the body depends on age, sex, weight, physical activities and environmental conditions such as weather.

In the Sirtfood Diet, water is a significant compound, for example, in fruits and beverages. Drinks such as unsweetened coffee-infused or flavored water are good options for staying hydrated.

Water provides a medium over all the physiological processes. Thus, frequent consumption of water and other drinks containing water like the ones included in the Sirtfood Diet reduces fatigue and boosts body energy.

Chapter 2.   Sirtfood Diet Health Benefits

There is proof that sirtuin activators provide a wide variety of health benefits like muscle strengthening and appetite suppression.

Or improved memory, better control of blood sugar level, and the clearance of damage caused by free radical molecules that build up in cells and result in cancer and other diseases.

"The positive effects of the intake of food and beverages rich in sirtuin activators in decreasing chronic diseases risks are an important observational evidence," said Professor Frank Hu, an authority on diet and epidemiology at Harvard University in a recent paper in Advanced Nutrition.

Losing weight is simply not enough nowadays, as the diet you have to follow needs to have plenty of health benefits as well; otherwise, you can't stick to it in the long run.

Therefore, you need to see the bigger picture and not focus on losing a lot of pounds in a very short amount of time.

Radical diets usually come with side effects, but if you find a meal plan that works for you in terms of weight loss and delivers plenty of health benefits, why not stick to it and make it your default diet?

The less processed food you eat, the more chances you will have to experience the health benefits from your meal plan, so you don't have to see a doctor very often.

Let's have a look in detail at the main benefits the Sirtfood Diet will guarantee you for a lifetime.

Immediate Weight Loss

The most obvious of the health benefit is that you will lose weight on this diet. Whether you are exercising or not, there is no way that you would not lose weight when you follow the diet to a T.

This diet will have you restrict your calories enough that anyone would lose weight. The average person uses around 2,000 calories per day; you will be providing yourself with 1,000 or 1,500 calories based on the phase that you are in.

Weight loss is caused by a calorie deficit — it is as simple as that. When you restrict your calories, but you keep your metabolism up, you will find that you will naturally lose weight.

This is normal. However, usually, that weight loss is a mix between fat and muscle. As you lose weight and muscle, you would then naturally see your metabolism slow as well.

Of course, this means that over time, your weight loss plan is not nearly as effective as it was supposed to be, and as a direct result, you will have to cut calories further to keep that deficit between consumed calories and the calories that your body naturally burns. This means that weight loss eventually slows, or even plateaus if all you do is make use of a weight-loss regimen through cutting calories. You will lose muscle if you are not careful with the weight loss regimen and that will work against you.

However, thanks to the fact that you do not lose muscle mass during the Sirtfood Diet, you do not have to worry about this problem; you simply continue to lose weight because you are able to maintain your metabolism at levels that will be favorable to you continuing to lose weight.

Sure enough, one remarkable observation of the Sirtfood Diet trial is that participants lost excessive weight while building muscle, contributing to a more toned body. It is the beauty of Sirtfoods: fat burning is activated, but muscle growth, maintenance and repair are promoted as well.

Positive Influence on Genetic

Is thinness is a genetic trait? And if so, how can you ever hope to lose weight?

Even if some people are blessed by activated "skinny genes" and can eat whatever they want without worrying about gaining weight, you can activate your skinny genes as well; they are inscribed in our DNA after all! We just need to remind our cells of that... It's not science fiction, our environment and our habits shape our cellular growth and gene replication: it's called epigenetic.

Every one of us has genes able to activate sirtuins, or SIRTs, they are metabolic regulators that control our ability to burn fat and cell regeneration. You can imagine them as sensors that get activated when our energy levels are low. That is the base of most fasting diets. But let's see some of the drawbacks of this type of diets.

Many fasting diets have become popular in the past years. The most well-known are the several variants of the intermittent fasting structure, such as the five-two diet. In the five-two diet, you fast during the weekend and eat normally during the working days of the week. These diets have proven and demonstrated effects on longevity, weight loss and overall health.

This is because these fasting diets activate the 'skinny gene' in our body. This gene causes the fat storage processes to shut down and for the body to enter a state of 'survival' mode, which in turn causes the body to burn fat.

Anytime cells in your body replicate there is a small chance of your DNA being damaged in the process. However, if your body repairs dying and older cells there is no risk of DNA damage, which is the reason why fasting is associated with lower prevalence of degenerative disease, such as Alzheimer's.

However, the problem with fasting diets, as the name implies, is that you have to fast. Fasting feels awful, especially when we are surrounded by other people having regular eating habits. It also puts some social spotlight on your own diet – explaining to your co-workers or your extended family why you are not eating on certain days is bound to generate incredulity and challenges to your diet regime.

Furthermore, even though fasting has numerous associated benefits, there are some downsides too. Fasting is associated with muscle loss, as the body doesn't discriminate between muscle mass and fat tissue when choosing cells to burn for energy.

Fasting also risks malnutrition, simply by not eating enough foods to get essential nutrients. This risk can be somewhat alleviated by taking vitamin supplements and eating nutrient rich foods, but fasting can also slow and halt the digestive system altogether – preventing the absorption of supplements. These supplements also need dietary fat to be dissolved, which you might also lack if you were to implement a strict fasting method.

On top of this, fasting isn't appropriate for a huge range of people. Obviously, you don't want children to fast and potentially inhibit their growth. Likewise, the elderly, the ill and pregnant women are all just too vulnerable to the risks of fasting.

Additionally, there are several psychological detriments to fasting, despite commonly being associated with spiritual revelations. Fasting makes you irritable and causes you to feel slightly on edge – your body is telling you constantly that you need to forage for food, enacting physical processes that affect your mood and emotions.

Sirtuins were first discovered in 1984 in yeast molecules. Of course, once it became apparent that sirtuin activators affected a variety of factors, such as lifespan and metabolic activity, interest in these proteins blossomed.

Sirtuin activators boost your mitochondria's activity, the part of the biological cell which is responsible for the production of energy. This in turn mirrors the energy-boosting effects which also occur due to exercise and fasting. The Sirtfood Diet is thought to start a process called adipogenesis, which prevents fat cells from duplicating – which should interest any potential dieter.

Diabetes

If you are suffering from diabetes, then you should know that activating sirtuins will make insulin work more effectively. Insulin is the hormone primarily responsible for controlling the levels of sugar in the blood. SIRT1 works perfectly with metformin (one of the most powerful antidiabetic drugs).

As it turns out, pharmaceutical companies are adding sirtuin activators to metformin treatments. These studies were conducted on animals, and the results were simply amazing. It was noticed that an 83 percent reduction of the metformin dose is required to achieve the same effects.

By increasing the amount of insulin that can be released, SIRT1 can help tackle diabetes by causing higher amounts of blood sugar to be converted into fat. So, as the key to both diabetes and weight gain is insulin resistance, there can be positive news for the waistline.

Cognitive Impairment and Alzheimer's

Sirtuins have been shown to have an impact: on neurodegenerative diseases that cause cognitive impairment like Alzheimer's disease.

This is because sirtuins help regulate appetite and manage other brain stimuli enhancing the communication signals in the brain itself, improving the cognitive function, and lowering brain inflammation.

Individuals with Alzheimer's have been found to have notably lower levels of sirtuins than healthy peers, although the mechanism of action between sirtuin and the disease is not fully known.

What is known is that the Sirtfood Diet helps prevent build-ups of amyloid-B and tau protein, molecules which are responsible for the plaques in the brains of people with Alzheimer's (and all the similar diseases that cause cognitive impairment).

Improved Energy

Eating food in frequent meals can help boosting vitality levels and giving the brain a steady supply of energy for all its functions.

As we will see later in the book, the Sirtfood Diet allows you to eat 5 times per day; juice, snack or meal depending on the phase of the diet you are in.

Frequent meals help control blood sugar and hunger throughout the day, having a positive effect on energy level too thanks to sirtuins effect. Sirtfoods that can be consumed frequently include coffee, soy, dark chocolate, and blueberries.

Consumption of food with a low glycemic index may assist in the reduction of the lag in energy that occurs after taking food with fast absorption of sugars and refined starches. Sirtfood promotes the inclusion of foods with low glycemic index like vegetables, nuts, and whole grains.

These foods improve the energy-boosting effect in the body.

Chapter 3.   Different Options for Every Need

The Sirtfood Diet, unlike fasting, doesn't involve skipping meals in order to experience the benefits it can offer. Therefore, you are not going through starvation to reach your weight loss and health goals. Nonetheless, the diet involves a very short period of caloric restriction that will require a bit of focus then you will increase calories again, going back to having breakfast, lunch, dinner, and snacks.

The Sirtfood Diet has been studied to meet the needs of the vast majority of people who need to lose weight.

Only people with serious illnesses, who are pregnant or breastfeeding should pay attention and skip to the maintenance phase, avoiding caloric restriction altogether. This means that they will still include healthy Sirtfoods (with their weight loss properties) in their everyday meals. They may not be able to take advantage of Phase 1 boost but still they will do the best choices for their health and weight loss.

Remember, even if you do not or cannot follow through with the restrictions, there is still a great benefit with adding the sirtuin-rich foods to your diet. As we will address shortly, many of the foods rich in sirtuins are highly nutritious and there is no doubt about the fact that they are very healthy and they should be included in your diet whether you want to follow the Sirtfood Diet or not.

Now you are probably wondering, "How am I going to lose pounds by eating three meals a day?"

The secret lies within the meal plan, as it can seriously deliver amazing results. Depending on the Phase you are in, you can enjoy eating dark chocolates and red wine while losing weight!

The average weight loss during the first week has been proved around seven pounds.

Of course not all bodies react the same to this diet, so the weight loss can be more or less visible but what this diet promises to deliver is that you will have outstanding results for trying it.

Once you are satisfied with the weight you reached, you can simply go into the maintenance phase of this diet and then transition to a normal healthy diet, still full of sirtuin-rich food. Sounds neat, right? This is what's great about this diet — it gives you the possibility to preserve your ideal weight long term, unlike many other radical diets where most people complain that they start to gain weight immediately after quitting.

Chapter 4.   The Sirtfood Diet Plan

The official Sirtfood Diet combines a short phase of calorie restriction with a long-term commitment to nutrient-dense sirtuin-activating foods. But before explaining how the diet is structured in detail, let's talk about two different and very important subjects when you are trying to achieve long lasting results.

The Difference between Diet and Dieting

How you eat every day is your "diet", restricting how you eat is "dieting".

Aside from the first week, Phase 1, the Sirtfood diet is not a traditional diet in that: instead of simply restricting calories, you focus on increasing nutrition and improving quality of the food you eat.

There are two main phases in the Sirtfood Diet, which take up 3 weeks and are designed to set the stage for incorporating sirtfoods into your lifelong diet, eliminating your need to ever resort to dieting again and a third phase dedicated to transition to a normal (not restricted) healthy sirtfood-rich diet.

The average American over-consumes solid fats and sugars, refined grains, sodium, and saturated fat. They also under-consume vegetables, fruits, whole grains, as well as the nationally recommended intake of dairy and oils.

If this sounds like it matches your current eating patterns, don't be too hard on yourself, you're certainly not alone. And you've been practically brainwashed into adopting these poor nutrition habits.

The number of fast-food restaurants continues to grow, as do options for pre-made, packaged foods full of empty calories and misleading promises.

When you live on a diet of these foods that are lacking nutrition for too long, you find yourself getting sick and overweight.

How many times have you found yourself dieting, starving yourself for weeks to lose 20 pounds? Maybe you've even been successful a time or two and lost weight, but within a few months, all the weight you lost had found its way home again, and brought a few extra friends along.

Studies show that when you restrict your calories severely for an extended period of time, you will gain the weight back as quickly as it came off, and you will do additional damage to your liver, kidneys and muscle mass as well. Short term calorie restriction, such as the first

Week 1: First 3 days will include 3 juices per day; remaining 4 days will include 2 juices per day.

Monday

Breakfast: Sirtfood Green juice

Snack: Two squares of dark chocolate

Lunch: Sirtfood Green juice

Snack: Sirtfood Green juice

Dinner: Sirtfood meal

Drink the juices at three distinct times of the day, like shown, in the morning as soon as you wake up, lunch, and mid-afternoon. For dinner choose a recipe in Appendix A.

Tuesday

Breakfast: Sirtfood Green juice

Snack: Two squares of dark chocolate

Lunch: Sirtfood Green juice

Snack: Sirtfood Green juice

Dinner: Sirtfood meal

The formula is identical to that of the first day, and the only thing that changes is the recipe for dinner, as usual selected from recipes in Appendix A.

Wednesday

Breakfast: Sirtfood Green juice

Snack: Two squares of dark chocolate

Lunch: Sirtfood Green juice

Snack: Sirtfood Green juice

Dinner: Sirtfood meal

This is the last day you will consume three green juices a day; tomorrow, you will switch to two. Take this opportunity to browse other drinks that you can have during the diet, such as coffee, green tea or herbal tea.

As usual, select your dinner from recipes in Appendix A.

Thursday

Breakfast: Sirtfood Green juice

Snack: Sirtfood Green juice

Lunch: Sirtfood meal

Snack: Two squares of dark chocolate.

Dinner: Sirtfood meal

The big change from the previous three days is that you will only drink two juices instead of three and that you will have two meals instead of one.

As usual, select your lunch and dinner from recipes in Appendix A.

Friday

Breakfast: Sirtfood Green juice

Snack: Sirtfood Green juice

Lunch: Sirtfood meal

Snack: Two squares of dark chocolate.

Dinner: Sirtfood meal

On the fifth day, you will intake 2 green juices and 2 meals.

As usual, select your lunch and dinner from recipes in Appendix A.

Saturday

Breakfast: Sirtfood Green juice

Snack: Sirtfood Green juice

Lunch: Sirtfood meal

Snack: Two squares of dark chocolate.

Dinner: Sirtfood meal

On the sixth day, you will assume 2 green juices and 2 meals

As usual, select your lunch and dinner from recipes in Appendix A.

Sunday

Breakfast: Sirtfood Green juice

Snack: Sirtfood Green juice

Lunch: Sirtfood meal

Snack: Two squares of dark chocolate.

Dinner: Sirtfood meal

On the seventh day, you will consume 2 green juices; 2 meals.

The seventh day is the last of phase 1 of the diet. Instead of considering it as an end, see it as a beginning, because you are about to embark on a new life, in which Sirtfoods will play a central role in your nutrition. Today's menu is a perfect example of how easy it is to integrate them in abundance into your daily diet.

As usual, select your lunch and dinner from recipes in Appendix A.

Notes.

It is suggested that you should also not consume any of your juices, or your main meal, after 7 pm. This is advised due to our natural circadian rhythm or our 'body clock 'and how it affects our body. Generally speaking, our body wants to prepare and burn energy in the morning, whilst store and retain energy during the evening. Therefore, if you eat later at night, you have a higher chance of energy in your food being stored as fat.

You should also feel free to drink non-calorie fluids. Whilst this technically does include calorie-free fizzy drinks, green tea, black coffee, and of course, water are better choices. One surprising finding is that small doses of lemon juice can prove helpful in increasing sirtuin absorption, so consider add a dash to your water or green tea.

Note that only black coffee is recommended; since milk, sugar, and sweeteners diminish the sirtuin absorption and interfering with the calorie count. Another caveat is that you shouldn't change your coffee consumption too much from your regular habits. A sudden drop in consumption will make you feel awful; a sharp increase will make you feel jittery. Change your coffee habits gradually.

Phase 2: Maintenance

Congratulations! You have finished the first "hardcore" week. The second phase – maintenance - is easier.

It will last two weeks and it will keep including sirtuin-filled food selections to your everyday meals.

Calorie intake for this phase is set to 1500 kcal. By doing so, your body will undergo the fat-burning stage and muscle gain plus a boost on your immune system and overall health.

For this phase, you can now have 3 balanced Sirtfood-filled meals each day plus 1 green juice a day.

Try choosing healthier alternatives with adding Sirtfood in each meal as much as possible.

You should consume the same beverages you were drinking in phase 1, with the slight change that you are welcome to enjoy the occasional glass of red wine (although don't drink more than 3 per week).

Monday to Sunday (week 2 and week 3)

Breakfast: Sirtfood meal

Snack: Sirtfood Green juice

Lunch: Sirtfood meal

Snack: Sirtfood snack or two squares of dark chocolate

Dinner: Sirtfood meal

As usual, select your lunch and dinner from recipes in Appendix A.

You may also add a glass of red wine per day if you feel to.

As far as drinks, you can have coffee, green tea and other no-calorie drinks on a daily basis.

Phase 3 – Transition to Normal Healthy Eating

After 2 weeks of mildly restricted calorie intake you are now ready to move back up to a regular calorie intake with the aim to keep your Sirtfood intake high. You should have experienced some degree of weight loss by now, but most of all, you should also feel fitter and re-invigorated.

Suggested meal plan is

Monday to Sunday

Breakfast: Sirtfood meal

Snack: Sirtfood Green juice or Sirtfood snack (one a day each)

Lunch: Sirtfood meal

Snack: Sirtfood Green juice or Sirtfood snack (one a day each)

Dinner: Sirtfood meal

Eating reasonable portions of balanced meals, you shouldn't feel hungry or be consuming too much. This is the main reason why Sirtfood Diet is very sustainable. After 3 weeks only you have changed your eating habits for the better, improving you way to nourish your body. Just keep going, without restricting portions as in the previous weeks and gradually implementing more and more sirtfoods into your lifestyle.

If you continuously try and withhold yourself from temptation and always moderate your eating habits, you are bound to crack and fall off the wagon sooner or later. Instead you should be combining your regular eating habits with the Sirtfood diet principles, slowly aligning your natural eating tendencies and taste with the Sirtfood ideal.

And remember, whenever you need a fat-burning boost, you can re-implement the three-phases of Sirtfood Diet to speed up your weight loss and cleanse your body.

Chapter 5. Sirtfood Ingredients

The Sirtfood Diet has some major advantages compared to other meal plans or programs designed to lose weight and get healthier. The ingredients are very familiar, and you can easily combine them with other healthy foods that are not rich in sirtuins.

Also, this diet is very permissive. You can try plenty of food out there, and you are not too limited to veggies and fruits.

There might be people trying sirtfoods and not losing weight. In this case, their problem lies within the form, variety, and quantity. It is very hard to have a meal consisting only of sirtfoods, so you need to find the right balance between sirtfoods and normal food.

Having regular meals is very important because if you don't have the meals within a set timeframe, the diet might not work. The general rule about not eating too much at dinner or having dinner late in the evening applies.

Throughout recent years there has been in several areas an increasing aversion to grains. Studies, however, link whole grain consumption with decreased inflammation, diabetes, heart disease, and cancer.

Although they do not equal the pseudo-grain buckwheat Sirtfood qualifications, we do see the existence of substantial sirtuin-activating nutrients in other whole grains. And needless to say, their sirtuin-activating nutrient quality is decimated when whole grains are converted into refined "clean" forms.

Such modified models are quite vulnerable groups and are interested in a number of state-of-the-art health problems. We're not saying you can never eat them, but instead, you're going to be much better off sticking to the whole-grain version whenever possible.

Now, let's try to understand the secret of these sirtfoods. What exactly do they contain that activates sirtuins?

Arugula contains nutrients like kaempferol and quercetin. Buckwheat contains rutting. Capers have the same nutrients as arugula. Celery has luteolin and apigenin. Cocoa contains epicatechin.

Chilies have a higher concentration of myricetin and luteolin. Coffee contains caffeic acid. Widely used in the Mediterranean diet, the extra-virgin olive oil has hydroxytyrosol and oleuropein. Kale contains the same nutrients as arugula and capers. You can find ajoene and myricetin in garlic.

In green tea, you can find EGCG epigallocatechin gallate. Medjool dates contain caffeic and Gallic acid. Parsley has myricetin and apigenin. In red endives, you can find luteolin. Quercetin can be found in red onions.

Strawberries contain fisetin. Walnuts are a great source of Gallic acid. Turmeric has cur cumin. Soy contains formononetin and daidzein. Red wine has piceatannol and resveratrol.

Indeed, they all have the power to trigger sirtuins, but as it turns out, a standard US diet is very poor when it comes to these nutrients. A proper Sirtfood Diet should allow you to consume hundreds of milligrams of these important ingredients per day. Obviously, if you manage to introduce most of the ingredients and sirtfoods mentioned above into your daily meal plan, you can effectively reap the benefits of this diet.

Are Supplements OK?

The nutrients mentioned above should be consumed in a natural state. This is how this diet works. You may not have the same effects if you take supplements, as the body absorbs and assimilates them a lot better in their natural form. If you take, for instance, resveratrol, this nutrient is poorly absorbed in a supplement form. However, if you consume it in a natural form, the absorption is six times higher.

There are many studies that suggest when certain vitamins, minerals, antioxidants or even polyphenols are isolated and consumed outside of their natural food source, they are not metabolized effectively and, in some cases, can even be detrimental to your health.

Humans are very impressive in the field of science and medicine, but nature has secrets we haven't even begun to unravel, so whenever possible, it's in your best interest to find the most natural source of nutrition as possible.

It is good to have as many of these sirtfoods as possible to make sure you are getting the necessary intake of sirtuin-activating nutrients. Most of them are very common or familiar, and this is the beauty of the Sirtfood diet: it is not something extraordinary to eat garlic or red onion, strawberries, blueberries, or walnuts. It is highly recommended to make sure you include turmeric in your diet, as well.

When it comes to consuming fruits and veggies, most nutritionists would agree that it is best to consume them fresh and raw. This is how you will get all the nutrients and vitamins from them.

However, when it comes to leafy greens, another way to reap all their benefits is juice them, as this procedure removes the low-nutrient fiber from them and allows you to have a super concentrated dose of sirtuin-activating polyphenols.

Since this diet allows you to eat plenty of foods, it rocks when it comes to diversity. This is why you can simply feel free to consume meat, fish, and seafood if you want. As a general rule of thumb, consume less red meat beef and pork and more poultry, fish, and seafood.

The Sirtfood diet should slowly become your default meal plan. Therefore, you don't have to stick just to the four-week meal plan. Sirtuins need to be in your diet every day of the week, so why stop after finishing the fourth week? If you have a good thing running, you really don't need to interrupt it. Plus, the longer you are following this diet, the more health benefits you will experience. This should be the ultimate motivation to make you try the Sirtfood diet on a regular basis. You need to check yourself whether or not you want to prevent or even reverse some of the most common diseases caused by poor diet, slow down your aging process, and lose some weight while doing it.

Note.

If your doctor or primary care physician has advised you to take a supplement, follow their advice. There are circumstances when supplementation is critical for your survival. There are many more circumstances when taking supplements is simply advisable.

Vegans, for example, are almost always deficient in vitamin B12 and Omega 3 fatty acids because both of those nutrients are most commonly found in fatty, oily fish. If following a completely plant-based diet is your ethical or moral choice, you may need to supplement for your best health.

20 Main Sirtfoods to Include In Your Everyday Meals

There are various foods that can be included in your plan of Sirtfood Diet. This chapter is all about the various types of sirtfoods that you should include in the diet for getting the best results.

The following twenty foods contain the highest amounts of sirtuin-activating polyphenols. The levels of polyphenol are not uniformly distributed in all these foods, and some of them contain higher amounts. Moreover, different types of polyphenols are present in each of them, and they are associated with special effects on the sirtuin gene.

This is why one of the most important aspects of the Sirtfood Diet is to use a variety of foods.

Each of these foods has their own impressive health qualities, but nothing compares to when they are combined.

Buckwheat

Flour that is made from buckwheat helps a lot in losing weight. The overall fat content of buckwheat is very low. In fact, the calorie count is less from normal rice or wheat. As the flour comes with a low amount of saturated form of fat, it can stop you from binge-eating or eating unnecessarily. So, it can help in facilitating and maintaining quick digestion. Because of the low amount of fat along with a greater quantity of minerals, it can facilitate controlling diabetes of type II.

Arugula

Arugula is a great sirtfood vegetable and is low in calories. It will not only help you to lose weight but also comes with several healthy properties. Arugula is rich in chlorophyll that can help in preventing DNA and liver damage resulting from aflatoxins. For getting the best from the arugula, it is always recommended to consume this vegetable raw. It is made of 95% water, and thus it can also act as a cooling and hydrating food for the summer days. Vitamin K plays an important role in maintaining bone health.

Capers

Caper is the unripe flower bud of Capparis spinosa. It is rich in compounds of flavonoid that also includes quercetin and rutin, great sources of antioxidants. Antioxidants can act readily in preventing free radicals that can lead to skin diseases and also cancer. Capers can help in keeping a check on diabetes. It contains several chemicals that can keep the level of blood sugar under control.

Chilies

Consumption of chilies in your daily diet can help in burning down calories. So, adding a bit of spice to your daily diet like cayenne or bird's eye chili can help in getting rid of the extra calories and help boosting up the metabolism. It also helps in lowering the levels of blood sugar. It has also been found that people who have the habit of consuming chili in their diet can feel full easily, and thus, it can lower your food cravings.

Celery

Celery contains very low calories and that is excellent for losing weight. It can also aid in preventing dehydration as it comes with a great amount of water and electrolytes that also helps in lowering bloating. It comes with antiseptic properties and prevents various problems of the kidney. Consumption of this vegetable can also help in excreting toxic elements from the body. Celery comes with great amounts of vitamin K and vitamin C, along with potassium and folate.

Cocoa

Intake of cocoa, even in its chocolate form, can help in controlling weight. Cocoa comes along with fat-burning properties and is the prime reason why most of the trainers suggest mixing cocoa in shakes before exercising. It can help in reducing inflammation and thus can also help in proper digestion. Cocoa is rich in antioxidants like polyphenols.

Coffee

Coffee is one of the most famous beverages that can be found all over the world. Coffee comes with a very low-calorie count. Caffeine is a form of natural stimulant that is abundant in coffee. It increases the mental functionality and alertness, making the brain alert and sharpened. Caffeine can help in improving metabolism and thus can act as a great weight loss component. But do not exceed as it can affect your sleeping patterns.

Olive Oil

Olive oil has always been popular for cooking food. Olive oil that is of the extra virgin category can help you in losing weight as it is unrefined and unprocessed. It comes with a great percentage of fatty acids of mono-saturated type that plays an important role in losing weight. Olive oil is also rich in vitamin E that is good for the health of hair and skin. It comes with great properties of anti-inflammation as well. Olive oil helps in aiding low absorption of fat and thus makes your food healthy and tasty at the same time.

Garlic

Garlic is one of those vegetables that can be found in every kitchen. Consumption of raw garlic can help in boosting energy levels that can aid in losing weight. Garlic is well known for suppressing appetite that can help you in staying full for more amount of time. Thus, with the consumption of garlic, you will be able to prevent yourself from overeating.

A strong relationship can be found between burning fat and the consumption of garlic. Garlic helps in stimulating the process of fat burning and also helps in removing harmful toxins from the body.

Green Tea

Green tea is often regarded as the healthiest type of beverage that can be found on this planet. This is mainly because green tea is full of antioxidants, along with several other plant compounds that can provide you with several health benefits like theine. Theine effect is similar to caffeine and acts as a stimulant for burning fat.

It can also help in boosting your levels of energy at the time of exercising. Green tea comes with a high concentration of minerals and vitamins, along with low content of calories. It can help in improving the metabolic rate as well.

Kale

Kale is a very popular vegetable that comes with excellent weight loss properties. It is a vegetable that is rich in antioxidants like vitamin C that performs various important functions in the body cells, along with improving the bone structure of the body.

It is rich in vitamin K and comes with excellent capabilities of binding calcium. Kale can provide you with 2.4 g of dietary fiber and thus can help in reducing the feeling of hunger. It comes with compounds rich in sulfur and can help in detoxifying the liver.

Medjool Dates

Dates are rich in dietary fibers along with fatty acids that can help in losing the extra kilos when consumed in moderation as they are very caloric. They help staying healthy and fit thanks to their protein content. Moderate consumption of dates daily can help in boosting the functioning of the immune system.

Parsley

Parsley is a very common herb that can be found in every kitchen. The leaves are rich in important compounds such as vitamin A, vitamin B, vitamin C, and vitamin K. Important minerals such as potassium and iron can also be found in parsley. As it acts as a natural form of diuretic, it can help in flushing out toxins along with any excess fluid. Parsley is rich in chlorophyll, and it can effectively aid in losing weight. It also helps in keeping the levels of blood sugar under control. Parsley comes with certain enzymes that can help in improving the process of digestion and also helps in weight loss.

Red Endive

Endives are rich in fiber with a low-calorie count. They are rich in fiber that can help in slowing down the process of digestion and keeps the level of energy stable, a great combination of elements that can help in promoting weight loss. Thanks to their water and fiber content, you will be able to consume more volume of food without the risk of consuming extra calories. It is rich in potassium and folate as well, important for the proper health of the heart. Potassium can act very well in lowering the level of blood pressure.

Red Onion

Red onion is rich in an antioxidant named quercetin. Red onions can help in adding extra flavor to your food without piling up extra calories. Quercetin helps in promoting burning down extra calories. It can also help in dealing with inflammation. Red onion is rich in fiber and thus can make you feel full for a long period without the urge to consume extra calories. It can also help in improving the level of blood sugar and can deal with diabetes of type II.

Soy

It has been found that increasing the consumption of soy can help in reducing your body weight thanks to its essential amino-acids. It is rich in fiber that can help you to stay full for long. Soy can also help in regulating the level of blood sugar and can have great control over the appetite. It can also promote better quality skin, hair, and nails, besides its weight loss benefits.

Red Wine

According to some recent studies, it has been found that drinking red wine in moderation can help in cutting down extra pounds. Red wine consists of a polyphenol named resveratrol that can aid in losing weight. This polyphenol can help in converting white fat, the larger cells that store up energy, into brown fat that can deal with obesity. It can also reduce the risk of heart attack. In fact, serious problems like Alzheimer's disease and dementia can also be reduced by consuming two glasses of red wine daily. Red wine can also prevent the development of type II diabetes.

Strawberries

Strawberries are filled with fiber, vitamins, polyphenols, zero cholesterol, and zero fat. They are also a great source of magnesium. Potassium and vitamin C. The high fiber content also assists in losing weight. It can help you in staying full that will reduce the chances of overeating or snacking. A hundred grams of strawberries comes with 33 calories only. Strawberries also help in improving the system of digestion and can also readily eliminate toxins from the body.

Turmeric

Turmeric is one of the primary spices in every household. It comes with an essential antioxidant called curcumin. It helps in dealing with obesity, disorders related to the stomach, and other health problems. It can help in reducing inflammation that is linked with obesity. Remember to add some pepper when using turmeric: the absorption of curcumin will be higher.

Walnuts

Walnuts are rich in healthy fats along with fiber that can aid in losing weight. They can provide you with a great deal of energy as well. They contain high quantities of PUFAs or polyunsaturated fats that can help in keeping the level of cholesterol under check while alpha-linolenic acid helps in burning body fat quickly and promotes proper heart health.

More Sirtfoods for your recipes

Besides the 20 main foods shown above, there are many other sirtfoods you can include in your meals, this will help you having a very colorful and varied diet which will aid fat burning and muscle gain thanks to sirtuin activation.

- Apples
- Artichokes
- Asparagus
- Blackberries
- Blackcurrants
- Blueberries
- Broad beans
- Broccoli
- Chestnuts
- Chia seeds
- Chickpeas
- Chicory
- Chili peppers
- Chives
- Corn
- Cranberries
- Dill
- Endive lettuce
- Ginger
- Goji berries
- Green beans
- Mint
- Oregano
- Pak choi
- Peanuts
- Pistachios
- Plums
- Quinoa
- Raspberries
- Red Grapes
- Sage
- Shallots
- Spinach
- Sunflower seeds
- Watercress
- White Onions

Chapter 6.   Sirtfood Diet and Movement

The Sirtfood Diet is about consuming certain products that are designed to promote sustainable weight loss and wellbeing by definition. But with the advantages that you see by practicing the plan, you can fall into the trap of feeling there's no need to exercise. This will be endorsed by many diet books, saying how ineffective exercise is compared with following the right diet for weight loss. And it's real; we can't outdo a bad diet.

Forget about weight loss for a second and just glance at the litany of positive health benefits correlated with it. These include reduced risk of cardiovascular disease, stroke, hypertension, type 2 diabetes, osteoporosis, obesity and cancer, and improved mood, sleep, confidence, and a sense of wellbeing.

While many of the benefits of being active are driven by switching on our sirtuin genes, eating Sirtfoods shouldn't be used as a reason to not engage in exercise. Instead, we should understand how active the ideal complement to our Sirtfood intake is. It activates optimum stimulation of the sirtuin, and all the advantages that it provides, just as expected by definition.

Exercise during phase 1

During phase 1, caloric intake is restricted ad set to 1,000. During this week and in this week only, you may decide to avoid exercise if you don't feel to. It' up to you. If you are already used to training, you may want to keep going, maybe with less intensity. If you never trained before, the suggestion is to listen to your body.

Always remember that there's no need to climb a mountain during phase 1, a brisk walk will be ok and this should be sustainable for everyone.

Exercise during phase 2 and 3

During phase 2 and 3 you will gradually return to a normal calorie intake and you should feel a lot more energized so, why not put the excess energy to good use?

Plenty of athletes from have tried this diet, so you can easily conclude that it works perfectly fine with training and workout. In order to maximize the fat-burning effect, workout while dieting is important, but it is up to you how intense you want to train.

Suggested effort and basic healthy habits

What we are talking about here is meeting 150-minute (2 hours and 30 minutes) government guidelines of moderate physical activity a week. A moderate job is the equivalent of a brisk walk.

But that doesn't have to be limited to this. Any sport or physical activity you love is fitting. Pleasure and exercise do not have to be mutually exclusive! So, their social aspect enriches squad or group sports even more.

It's also about everyday things like taking the bike instead of the car, or getting off the bus one stop earlier, or just parking farther away to increase the distance you've got to walk around.

Take the stairs and not the lift.

Go outdoors and do gardening. Play in the park with your kids or get more out with the dog. Everything counts.

Everything that has you up and moving will activate your sirtuin genes regularly and at moderate intensity, enhancing the benefits of the Sirtfood Diet.

Chapter 7. Conclusion

Thank you for making it to the end!

As learned in the book, the key to a successful result is getting your body in perfect balance with a diet that's sustainable and providing all the nutrients we need that enhance our health.

It's about keeping on reaping the Sirtfood Diet's weight-loss rewards using the very best foods nature has to offer while getting pleasure and enjoyment from meals that include the higher the range of sirtuin-activating items possible and our favorite foods.

Keep following the simple rules in this book to maintain your results and live a healthy, happy life!

Appendix A – Sirtfood Recipes Ideas

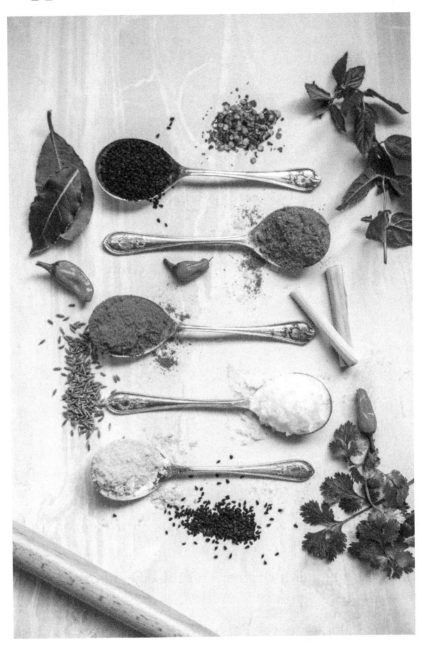

Breakfast

Sirtfood Green Juice

Preparation Time: 5 minutes

Number of Servings: 1

Ingredients:

Recipe 1:

1 tbsp. parsley

1 stalk celery

1 apple

½ lemon

Recipe 2:

1 cucumber

1 stalk celery

1 apple

3 mint leaves

Directions:

Choose one of the recipes above.

Add all ingredients into a juicer and extract the juice according to the manufacturer's method.

In case you don't have one, add all the ingredients in a blender and pulse until well combined.

Filter the juice through a fine mesh strainer and transfer into a glass. Top with water if needed. Serve immediately.

Avg. Nutrition Facts: Calories 30kcal, Fat 0.4 g, Carbohydrate 4.5 g, Protein 1 g

Pancakes with Caramelized Strawberries

Preparation time: 5 minutes

Cooking time: 15 minutes

Servings: 2

Ingredients:

1 egg

1 ½ oz. self-raising flour

1 ½ oz. buckwheat flour

1/3 cup skimmed milk

1 cup strawberries

2 tsp honey

Directions:

Mix the flours in a bowl; add the yolk and a bit of mix in a very thick batter. Keep adding the milk bit by bit to avoid lumps.

In another bowl, beat the egg white until stiff and then mix it carefully to the batter.

Put enough batter to make a 5-inch round pancake to cook 2 minutes per side until done. Repeat until all the pancakes are ready.

Put strawberries and honey in a hot pan until caramelized, the put half on top of each serving.

Nutrition Facts: Calories: 272, Fat: 4.3g, Carbohydrate: 26.8g, Protein: 23.6g

Scrambled Eggs and Red Onion

Preparation time: 2 minutes

Cooking time: 2 minutes

Servings: 1

Ingredients:

2 Eggs

1 tbsp. Parmesan

Salt and pepper

½ cup red onion

1 tbsp. parsley, finely chopped

Directions:

Put eggs and cheese with a pinch of salt and pepper and finely chopped onion in a bowl. Whisk quickly.

Cook the scrambled eggs in a skillet for 2 minutes, stirring continuously until done.

Nutrition Facts: Calories: 278, Fat: 5.4g, Carbohydrate: 12.8g, Protein: 18.9g

Matcha Overnight Oats

Preparation time: 10 minutes + overnight rest

Cooking time: 0 minutes

Servings: 2

Ingredients:

2 tsp. Chia seeds

3 oz. Rolled oats

1 tsp. Matcha powder

1 tsp Honey

1 ½ cups Almond milk

2 pinches Ground cinnamon

1 Apple, peeled, cored and chopped

4 walnuts

Directions:

Place the chia seeds and the oats in a container or bowl.

In a different jug or bowl, add the matcha powder and one tablespoon of almond milk and whisk with a hand-held mixer until you get a smooth paste, then add the rest of the milk and mix thoroughly.

Pour the milk mixture over the oats, add the honey and cinnamon, and then stir well. Cover the bowl with a lid and place in the fridge overnight.

When you want to eat, transfer the oats to two serving bowls, then top with the walnuts, and chopped apple.

Nutrition Facts: Calories 324, Carbs37 g, Fat14 g, Protein: 22g

Lunch/Dinner Recipes

Salmon Fritters

Preparation time: 10 minutes

Cooking time: 20 minutes

Servings: 2

Ingredients:

6 oz. salmon, canned

1 tbsp. flour

1 clove garlic, crushed

½ red onion, finely chopped

2 eggs

2 tsp. olive oil

Salt and pepper to taste

2 cups arugula

Directions:

Separate egg whites from yolks and beat them until very stiff. In a separate bowl mix salmon, flour, salt, pepper, onion, garlic, onion and yolks.

Add egg whites and slowly mix them together. Heat a pan on medium high. Add 1tsp. oil and when hot form salmon fritters with a spoon.

Cook until brown (around 4 minutes per side) and serve with arugula salad seasoned with salt, pepper and 1 tsp. olive oil.

Nutrition Facts: Calories: 320 Carbs: 18g Fat: 7g Protein: 27g

Mince Stuffed Eggplants

Preparation Time: 10 minutes

Cooking Time: 70 minutes

Servings: 6

Ingredients:

4 oz. lean mince

6 large eggplants

1 egg

3 tbsp. dry red wine

½ cup cheddar, grated

Salt and pepper, to taste

1 red onion

2 tsp. olive oil

2 tbsp. tomato sauce

2 tbsp. parsley

Directions:

Preheat oven to 350°F. Meanwhile, slice eggplants in 2 and scoop out the center part, leaving ½ inch of meat. . Place eggplants in a microwavable dish with about ½" of water in the bottom. Microwave on high for 4 minutes. In a saucepan, fry mince with onion for 5 minutes. Add wine and let evaporate. Add tomato sauce, salt, pepper, eggplant meat and cook around 20 minutes until done.

Combine, mince sauce, cheese, egg, parsley, salt and pepper in a large bowl and mix well. Pack firmly into eggplants. Return eggplants to the dish you first microwaved them in and bake for 25 to 30 minutes, or until lightly browned on top.

Nutrition Facts: Calories: 350 Carbs: 22g Fat: 10g Protein: 17g

Easy Shrimp Salad

Preparation time: 5 minutes

Cooking time: 0 minutes

Servings: 2

Ingredients:

2 cups red endive, finely sliced

1 cup cherry tomatoes, halved

1 tsp. of extra virgin olive oil

1 tbsp. parsley, chopped

3 oz. celery, sliced

6 walnuts, chopped

2 oz. red onion-sliced

1 cup yellow pepper, cubed

½ lemon, juiced

6 oz. steamed shrimps

Directions:

Put red endive on a large plate. Evenly distribute on top finely sliced onion, yellow pepper, cherry tomatoes walnuts, celery and parsley.

Mix oil, lemon juice with a pinch of salt and pepper and distribute the dressing on top.

Nutrition Facts: Calories: 353, Fat: 4.8g, Carbohydrate: 28.1g, Protein: 28.3g

Red Onion Frittata with Chili Grilled Zucchini

Preparation time: 5 minutes

Cooking time: 30 minutes

Servings: 2

Ingredients:

1 ½ cups red onion, finely sliced

3 eggs

3 oz. cheddar cheese

2 tbsp. milk

2 zucchini

2 tbsp. oil

1 clove garlic, crushed

½ chili, finely sliced

1 tsp. white vinegar

Salt and pepper to taste

Directions:

Heat the oven to 350°F. Cut the zucchini into thin slices; grill them and set them aside.

Add 3 eggs, shredded cheddar cheese, milk, salt, pepper, whisk well and pour in a silicone baking tray and cook 25-30 minutes in the oven. Mix garlic, oil, salt, pepper and vinegar and pour the dressing on the zucchini. Serve the frittata alongside the zucchini.

Nutrition Facts: Calories: 359, Fat: 7.8g, Carbohydrate: 18.1g, Protein: 21.3g

Garlic Chicken Burgers

Preparation time: 10 minutes

Cooking time: 10 minutes

Servings: 2

Ingredients:

8 oz. chicken mince

¼ red onion, finely chopped

1 clove garlic, crushed

1 handful of parsley, finely chopped

1 cup arugula

½ orange, chopped

1 cup cherry tomatoes

3 tsp extra virgin olive oil

Directions:

Put chicken mince, onion, garlic, parsley, salt pepper in a bowl and mix well. Form 2 patties and let rest 5 minutes.

Heat a pan with olive oil and when very hot cook 3 minutes per part.

They are also very good when grilled, if you opt for grilling; just brush the patties with a bit of oil right before cooking.

Put the arugula on two plates; add cherry tomatoes and orange on top, dress with salt and the remaining olive oil. Put the patties on top and serve.

Nutrition Facts: Calories: 353, Fat: 4.8g, Carbohydrate: 28.1g, Protein: 28.3g

Turmeric Turkey Breast with Cauliflower Rice

Preparation Time: 5 Minutes

Cooking time: 25 Minutes

Servings: 2

Ingredients:

2 cups cauliflower, grated

8 oz. turkey breast, cut in slices

2 tsp. ground turmeric

1/2 pepper, chopped

1/2 red onion, sliced

2 tsp. extra virgin olive oil

1 large tomato

1 clove garlic, crushed

1 cup milk, skimmed

2 tsp. buckwheat flour

1 oz. parsley, finely chopped

Directions:

Coat turkey slices with flour. Heat a pan on medium high with half the oil and when hot add the turkey. Let the meat color on all sides, then add milk, salt, pepper, 1 tsp. turmeric. Cook 10 minutes until the turkey is soft and the sauce has become creamy.

In a different pan, add the remaining oil and heat on medium heat. Add pepper, onion and tomato, 1 tsp. turmeric and let cook 3 minutes. Add the cauliflower and cook another 2 minutes. Add salt, pepper and let rest 2 minutes.

Serve the turkey with the cauliflower rice.

Nutrition Facts: Calories 107 Total Fat 2.9 g Total Carbs 20.6 g Protein 2.1 g

Mustard Salmon with Baby Carrots

Preparation Time: 10 Minutes

Cooking time: 40 Minutes

Servings: 2

8 oz. salmon fillet

2 tbsp. mustard

1 tbsp. white vinegar

1 tsp parsley, finely chopped

2 cups baby carrots

4 oz. buckwheat

2 tsp. extra virgin olive oil

Salt and pepper to taste

Directions:

Heat the oven to 400°F.

Boil the buckwheat in salted water for 25 minutes then drain. Dress with 1 tsp olive oil. Set aside. Put the salmon over aluminum foil.

Mix mustard and vinegar in a small bowl and brush the mixture over the salmon, close the foil in a packet. Cook in the oven 35minutes.

While the salmon is cooking, steam baby carrots for 6 minutes then put them in a pan on medium heat with 1tsp. olive oil, salt and pepper until light brown.

Serve the salmon with baby carrots and buckwheat on the side.

Nutrition Facts: Calories 314, Fat 9.1g, Protein 41.5g, Carbohydrate 15.7g

Turmeric Cous Cous with Edamame Beans

Preparation Time: 10 Minutes

Cooking time: 15 Minutes

Servings: 2

½ yellow pepper, cubed

½ red pepper, cubed

1 tbsp. turmeric

½ cup red onion, finely sliced

¼ cup cherry tomatoes, chopped

2 tbsp. parsley, finely chopped

5 oz. cous cous

2 tsp. extra virgin olive oil

½ eggplant

1 ½ edamame beans

Directions:

Steam edamame for 5 minutes and set aside. Add 6 oz. salted boiling water to cous cous and let rest until it absorbs the water.

In the meantime, heat a pan on medium high heat. Add oil, eggplant, peppers, onion and tomatoes, turmeric, salt and pepper. Cook for 5 minutes on high heat. Add the cous cous and edamame. Garnish with fresh parsley and serve.

Nutrition Facts: Calories 342, Carbs 15 g, Fat 5 g, Protein: 32g

Kale Omelette

Preparation time: 5 minutes

Cooking time: 5 minutes

Servings: 1

Ingredients:

2 Eggs

Garlic – 1 small glove

Kale – 2 handfuls

Goat cheese or

Sliced onion – ¼ cup

Extra virgin olive oil – 2 teaspoons

Directions:

Mince the garlic, and finely shred the kale. Break the eggs into a bowl, add a pinch of salt. Beat until well combined. Place a pan to heat over medium heat. Add one teaspoon of olive oil, add the onion and kale, cook for approx. Five minutes, or until the onion has softened and the kale is wilted. Add the garlic and cook for another two minutes.

Add one teaspoon of olive oil into the egg mixture, mix and add into the pan. Use your spatula to move the cooked egg toward the center and move the pan so that the uncooked egg mixture goes towards the edges.

Add the cheese into the pan just before the egg is fully cooked, then leave for a minute.

Serve immediately.

Nutrition Facts: Calories 219, Total Fat 18.6 g, Carbohydrate 7.7g, Protein 8.2g

Chocolate Dessert with Dates and Walnuts

Preparation Time: 10 Minutes

Cooking time: 15 Minutes

Servings: 2

Ingredients:

4 Medjool dates, pitted

2 tbsp. cocoa powder

1 cup milk, skimmed

1 tsp. agar powder

1 tbsp. peanut butter

1 pinch of salt

½ tsp. cinnamon

2 walnuts

1 tsp whole wheat flour

Directions:

Blitz dates, peanut butter and 1tbsp. milk in a food processor.

Put the mix in a pan; add cocoa, cinnamon, salt, flour, agar powder. Add the remaining hot milk bit by bit and mix well to obtain a smooth mixture. Turn the heat on, bring to a boil and cook around 6-8 minutes until dense. Divide in 2 cups, let cool and put in the fridge. Add chopped walnuts before serving.

Nutrition Facts: Calories 326, Carbs7 g, Protein: 25g, Fat3 g

Celery and Raisins Snack Salad

Preparation time: 10 minutes

Cooking time: 0 minutes

Servings: 4

Ingredients:

½ cup raisins

4 cups celery, sliced

¼ cup parsley, chopped

½ cup walnuts, chopped

Juice of ½ lemon

2 tbsp. extra virgin olive oil

Salt and black pepper to the taste

Directions:

In a salad bowl, mix celery with raisins, walnuts, parsley, lemon juice, oil, and black pepper, toss, divide into small cups and serve as a snack.

Nutrition Facts: Calories 120 Fat 1g Carbohydrate 6 g Protein 5 g

Dijon Celery Salad

Preparation time: 10 minutes

Cooking time: 0 minutes

Servings: 4

Ingredients:

2 tsp. honey

½ lemon, juiced

1 tbsp. Dijon mustard

2 tsp. extra virgin olive oil

Black pepper to taste

2 apples, cored, peeled and cubed

1 bunch celery roughly chopped

¾ cup walnuts, chopped

Directions:

In a salad bowl, mix celery and its leaves with apple pieces and walnuts.

Add black pepper, lemon juice, mustard, honey, and olive oil, whisk well, add to your salad, toss, divide into small cups and serve as a snack.

Nutrition Facts: Calories 125 Fat 2 Carbohydrate 7 g Protein 7 g

Mediterranean Tofu Scramble Snack

Preparation Time: 10 minutes

Cooking Time: 8 minutes

Servings: 2

Ingredients:

1 tsp. extra virgin olive oil

½ onion, chopped

½ zucchini, chopped

1 cup baby spinach

½ cup halved cherry tomatoes

1 tbsp. sundried tomatoes in oil

4 oz. tofu crumbled

Directions:

Place a pan on medium to low heat. Add oil. When the oil is hot, add all vegetables until they are soft. Season with salt and pepper and cook for 5 minutes.

Add spinach along with tomatoes and cook for a few minutes until the spinach wilts. Add tofu and mix well. Heat thoroughly. Adjust the seasoning if necessary. Remove from heat and serve as snack.

Nutrition Facts: Cal 134 Fat 9 g Carbs 5 g Fiber 1 g Protein 10 g

Appendix B – The Science behind the Sirtfood Diet

The Sirtfood Diet lays on a very strong scientific foundation. But that is exactly what the Sirtfood diet offers. Let's take a look at the science; I swear you won't get bored!

Scientific Studies on Skinny Gene

Many studies have indicated that weight variation is highly caused by genetics.

Nowadays, lots of researches have focused on people that are obese. A study was conducted by Professor Farooqi and his team to examine the real reason behind why some people remain thin and others do not.

The study comprises 14,000 participants out of whom there were 1,622 thin men and women 1,985 obese people and over 10,000 people with normal weight. The DNA of these people was compared. So, why studying the genes for this?

The truth is our DNA consists of proteins that are responsible for some particular functions in our body system. Any kind of change in this gene called genetic variant, can form another kind of protein and thus, altering the function of the protein within the body.

If it's a protein that involves in metabolism, there will be changes in the way our body processes and digests food and even stores them.

Going further, the team was able to identify some genetic variants that have the ability to increase people's risk of being obese. They were also able to find a novel genetic region that explains why some people are thin (Riveros-McKay et al. 2019).

The impact these genetic variants have on individual's weight were created in a risk score. It was discovered that thin individuals have a significantly low genetic risk score. The result proved that thin individuals are thin because they possess a lower genes burden that decreases a person's chance of being obese or overweight and not because they were created perfectly.

The belief of people for the past few years is that genetic is a causal factor of most diseases like cancer, obesity and so on.

Scientifically, genetics play just 10 percent roles in the risk of these diseases while the remaining 90 percent is dependent on environmental factors. Surprised right?

The way we sleep, eat, walk, behave, drink, reason and talk are all your environmental factors that you have control over.

In older adults, weight gain is a major determinant of how quickly they are aging. The fact that your body functions with the 90/10 rule makes it even easier for you to make good use of the genes at your disposal.

There are some genes called famine. These are genes that work to assist you extract as much energy as they can from the food you consume. Thereby, giving you the ability to store fat and live through famine.

You could have called this a brilliant idea some years back unlike now that these same genes can add to your weight. Although, 75 genes play a major role in becoming obese, there are major ones that can increase your risk of obesity and weight gain.

There are also ways in which you can control these genes and activate them as you wish. Not minding the fact that these genes are a part of you, there are ways you can control them, you have the power to decide how they interact and relate within your body.

Genes Associated with Weight Gain

There are certain genes that are associated with weight again which are responsible for how people gain weight unnecessarily mainly because of their eating habit. Some of these genes include:

FTO gene

This is the gene that has the strongest link with your body mass index. It's your greatest risk of diabetes and obesity. There's a variant that switches on the gene and if this variant is present in your body, you will not be able to control the hormone of satiety called leptin. Thus, making you to eat unnecessarily. The FTO gene acts like a fat sensor and people with this kind of gene tend to eat excessively most especially fatty foods, particularly in childhood. People who share an abnormal gene from the two parents weigh more and are at the greater risk of becoming obese. While people with normal gene have a lower risk of obesity.

The FTO gene can be switch on with adequate and proper physical exercise. Making sure you sleep between 7 to 8 hours at night, consuming low carbohydrates food and increasing your higher fiber intake. With proper dietary and good lifestyle, your risk of obesity can be reduced.

Melanocortin 4 Receptor

People born with this gene will consume more of snacks even if they are not hungry. They spend much of their time eating between meals, snacking on cake, chips and so on. This gene increases the urge for fat.

If you have an increasing urge for snack, simply learn to eat three times daily. Eat at intervals of four to six hours between each meal, with no snacking in between. Don't rush when eating. Set a boundary for your food consumption so you can easily combat the food addiction.

Adrenergic beta-2 Surface Receptor

This is a different kind of famine and it's associated with the distribution of fat. When this gene is turn on, the gene can hinder your body fat from breaking down, resulting in slower metabolic rate thus, making you store fat. This famine gene can increase your risk of obesity three times over. It can also increase the risk of type 2 diabetes. Also, people with this kind of gene find it really difficult to lose weight.

How do you deal with this gene? It's simple. Exercise is one of the possible solutions. Accept the fact that losing weight will be difficult for you so, don't feel bad when you see another person losing weight better and faster than you. Be disciplined in your eating habit. Eat the right kind of food with the right amount of nutrients. This is a slow and steady mission so you mustn't rush it.

Weight Loss Regulation

Furthermore, hypothalamic SIRT1 has been proven to help in weight loss. The hypothalamus is the central weight and energy balance controller. It modulates energy intake and energy consumption by neural inputs from the periphery as well as direct humor inputs, which senses the energy status of the body.

An adipokine, leptin, is one of the factors that signal that sufficient energy is stored on the periphery. Leptin plasma levels are favorable for adiposity, suppressing energy intake, and stimulating energy spending.

A prolonged increase in the level of plasma leptin in obese can cause leptin resistance. Leptin resistance, in turn, can affect the hypothalamus from having access to leptin, which also reduces leptin signals transduction in the hypothalamic neurons.

Reduced peripheral energy-sensing by leptin can lead to a positive energy balance and incremental weight gain and adiposity improvements, which further exacerbate leptin resistance.

Leptin resistance causes an increase in adiposity, just like weight gain are all associated with ageing. Similar observations occur in central insulin resistance. The improvement of the action of humoral factors in the hypothalamus can, therefore, prevent progressive weight gains, especially among middle-aged individuals.

SIRT1 is a protein deacetylase, NAD+ dependent that has many substrates, such as transcription factors, histones, co-factors, and various enzymes. SIRT1 improves the sensitivity to leptin and insulin by decreasing the levels of several molecules that impair the transduction of leptin and insulin signals. The hypothalamic SIRT1 and NAD+ levels decrease with age.

Increased in the level of SIRT1 has shown to improve kept in level in mice and so prevents age-related weight gain. By preventing the loss of age dependent SIRT1 hypothalamus role, there will be a boost in the activity of humoral factors in the hypothalamus and the central energy balance control.

Sirtuins and Metabolic Activity

SIRT1, just like other SIRTUINS family, is protein NAD+ dependent deacetylases that are associated with cellular metabolism. All sirtuins, including SIRT1 important for sensing energy status and in protection against metabolic stress. They coordinate cellular response towards Caloric Restriction (CR) in an organism. SIRT1 diverse location and allows cells to easily sense changes in the level of energy anywhere in the mitochondria, nucleus, and cytoplasm. Associated with metabolic health through deacetylation of several target proteins such as muscles, liver, endothelium, heart, and adipose tissue.

SIRT1, SIRT6, and SIRT7 are localized in the nucleus where they take part in the deacetylation of customers to influence gene expression epigenetically. SIRT2 is located in the cytosol, while SIRT3, SIRT4, and SIRT5 are located in the mitochondria where they regulate metabolic enzyme activities as well as moderate oxidative stress.

SIRT1, as most studies with regards to metabolism, aid in mediating the physiological adaptation to diets. Several studies have shown the impact of sirtuins on Caloric Restriction. Sirtuins deacetylase non-histone proteins that define pathways involved during the metabolic adaptation when there are metabolic restrictions. Caloric Restriction, on the other hand, causes the induction of expression of SIRT1 in humans. Mutations that lead to loss of function in some sirtuins genes can lead to a reduction in the outputs of caloric restrictions. Therefore, sirtuins have the following metabolic function:

Regulation in the liver

The Liver regulates the body glucose homeostasis. During fasting or caloric restriction, glucose level becomes low, resulting in a sudden shift in hepatic metabolism to glycogen breakdown and then to gluconeogenesis to maintain glucose supply as well as ketone body production to mediate the deficit in energy.

Also, during caloric restriction or fasting, there is muscle activation and liver oxidation of fatty acids produced during lipolysis in white adipose tissue. For this switch to occur, there are several transcription factors involved to adapt to energy deprivation. SIRT1 intervenes during the metabolic switch to see the energy deficit.

At the initial stage of the fasting that is the post glycogen breakdown phase, there is the production of glucagon by the pancreatic alpha cells to active gluconeogenesis in the Liver through the cyclic amp response element-binding protein (CREB), and CREB regulated transcription coactivator 2 (CRTC2), the coactivator.

Is the fasting gets prolonged, the effect is cancelled out and is being replaced by SIRT1 mediated CRTC2 deacetylase resulting in targeting of the coactivator for ubiquitin/ proteasome-mediated destruction?

SIRT1, on the other hand, initiates the next stage of gluconeogenesis through acetylation and activation of peroxisome proliferator-activated receptor coactivator one alpha, which is the coactivator necessary for fork head box O1. In addition to the ability of SIRT1 to support gluconeogenesis, coactivator one alpha is required during the mitochondrial biogenesis necessary for the liver to accommodate the reduction in energy status. SIRT1 also activates fatty acid oxidation through deacetylation and activation of the nuclear receptor to increase energy production.

SIRT1, when involved in acetylation and repression of glycolytic enzymes such as phosphoglycerate mutate 1 can lead to shutting down of the production of energy through glycolysis. SIRT6, on the other hand, can be served as a co-repressor for hypoxia-inducible Factor 1 Alpha to repress glycolysis. Since SIRT6 can transcriptionally be induced by SIRT1, sirtuins can coordinate the duration of time for each fasting phase.

Aside from glucose homeostasis, the liver also overtakes in lipid and cholesterol homeostasis during fasting. When there are caloric restrictions, the synthesis of fat and cholesterol in the liver is turned off, while lipolysis in the white adipose tissue commences.

The SIRT1, upon fasting, causes acetylation of steroid regulatory element-binding protein (SREBP) and targets the protein to destroy the ubiquitin-professor system.

The result is that fat cholesterol synthesis will repress. During the regulation of cholesterol homeostasis, SIRT1 regulates oxysterol receptor, thereby, assisting the reversal of cholesterol transport from peripheral tissue through upregulation of the oxysterol receptor target gene ATP-binding cassette transporter A1 (ABCA1).

Further modulation of the cholesterol regulatory loop can be achieved via bile acid receptor, that's necessary for the biosynthesis of cholesterol catabolic and bile acid pathways. SIRT6 also participates in the regulation of cholesterol levels by repressing the expression and post-translational cleavage of SREBP1/2, into the active form. Furthermore, in the circadian regulation of metabolism, SIRT1 participates through the regulation of cell circadian clock.

Mitochondrial SIRT3 is crucial in the oxidation of fatty acid in mitochondria. Fasting or caloric restrictions can result in up-regulation of activities and levels of SIRT3 to aid fatty acid oxidation through deacetylation of long-chain specific acyl-CoA dehydrogenase. SIRT3 can also cause activation of ketogenesis and the urea cycle in the liver.

SIRT1 also Add it in the metabolic regulation in the muscle and white adipose tissue. Fasting causes an increase in the level of SIRT1, leading to deacetylation of coactivator one alpha, which in turn causes genes responsible for fat oxidation to get activated.

The reduction in energy level also activates AMPK, which will activate the expression of coactivator one alpha. The combined effects of the two processes will give rise to increased mitochondrial biogenesis together with fatty acid oxidation in the muscle.

Sirtuins, Muscles and Oxidative Capacity

The expression of sirtuin in the muscle is affected by physical exercise that controls changes in the cellular antioxidant system, mitochondrial biogenesis, and oxidative metabolism.

Skeletal muscles are not only involved in force and movement but also involved in endocrine activities by its ability to secrete cytokines and transcription factors into the bloodstream, thereby, controls the function of other organs. Furthermore, skeletal muscle is a metabolically active tissue that plays a vital role in maintaining the metabolism of the body.

The skeletal muscle contains about 40% of the entire body weight. The insulin-stimulated uptake of glucose and the main energy-consuming lipid catabolism is mainly at this site. For the skeletal muscle, metabolic flexibility is essential to preserve physiological processes and metabolic homeostasis.

It determines the ability to switch from glucose to lipid oxidation. Advances in the understanding of the molecular mechanisms underlying skeletal muscle activity are a therapeutic benefit. Sirtuins' roles have been widely investigated in the skeletal muscle concerning their role in controlling glucose and lipid metabolism, insulin functions and sensitivity as well as function, and mitochondrial biogenesis.

Cellular metabolic stress results from physical exercise, which affects the sirtuins. The most studies sirtuins with this respect are SIRT1 and SIRT3, SIRT1 localized in the nucleus while SIRT3, in the mitochondria. SIRT3 is more expressed in type I muscle fiber.

A research conducted showed that mouse skeletal muscle SIRT3 reacted to the six weeks voluntary exercise dynamically to coordinate the downstream molecular response (Palacios et al., 2009). The result also showed that exercise causes an increase in SIRT3 protein, CREB, coactivator one alpha, and citrate synthesis activity.

The downregulation of CREB, AMP-activated protein kinase (AMPK) phosphorylation and the mRNA of PGC-1α are all symptoms of SIRT3 knockout. Showing that for SIRT3 to carry out the biological signals effectively, these key cellular molecules are essential.

Palacios et al. discovered that SIRT3 responds to exercise dynamically to enhance muscular energy homeostasis through AMPK and PGC-1α. Voluntary exercise causes an increase in the SIRT3 content of skeletal muscle. Muscle Immobility can, therefore, lead to the downregulation of SIRT3.

Furthermore, SIRT1 protein content and PGC-1 in the muscle tends to increase with exercise. Bayod et al. (2012) reported that SIRT1 protein content, as well as PGC-1 in rat's muscle, increased after 36 weeks of treadmill training together with enhancement in antioxidant defenses.

During exercise, there's an increase in demand for ATP, which in turn leads to increased NAD+ level and NAD+/NADH ratio. The result is an increase in the substrate for SIRT1 and SIRT3. SIRT3 is responsible for the increased ATP production as well as a reduction in protein synthesis in the mitochondria.

The ATP produced activates and deacetylases tricarboxylic acid (TCA) enzymes, electron transport chain, and β-oxidation, which maximizes the availability of reducing equivalents for ATP production. SIRT1, on the other hand, responds to exercise by contributing towards mitochondrial biogenesis via independent mechanism and PGC1α-dependent.

In summary, strenuous exercises activate SIRT1, which enhances biogenesis and mitochondrial oxidative capacity.

Then, having several sessions of exercise will activate both SIRT1 and also SIRT3, which in turn activate ATP production as well as the mitochondrial antioxidant function.

Sirtfood Diet Meal Plan

A Smart 4-Week Program To Jumpstart Your Weight Loss And Organize Your Meals Including The Foods You Love. Save Time, Feel Satisfied And Reboot Your Metabolism In One Month.

Kate Hamilton

Introduction

So, you are ready to lose weight, but you are not sure how. You are looking through diets online. You see the Mediterranean Diet. You see the Keto Diet. You see the Paleo Diet. There are countless options out there, all claiming that they are the best because they will help you to lose weight quickly.

Which one do you choose? You may scroll through them all without choosing one that seems right for you because you cannot think of one that is just right. You see all sorts of options, but none of them call out.

Maybe you've tried Keto, but you missed your fruits and carbs too much. Perhaps you tried the Paleo diet, but it just was not ok for you. Whether you have failed a diet in the past does not define your future: you can lose weight for good. You can learn how you can properly shed it off so that you will be able to love your own skin and stay healthier. You just need a new way of making it work for you.

The Sirtfood Diet was designed in the UK, by celebrities nutritionists, Aidan Goggins and Glen Matten, to include certain foods that help people rapidly shed pounds without the same consequences that are commonly seen in other diets.

Some diets require you to starve yourself, causing loss of muscle along with the fat. Others require you to give up on foods that you enjoy, making them so restrictive that they are difficult for most people to keep up with. In fact, the Sirtfood Diet encourages you to focus on sirtuin-rich foods that can be combined into delicious and satisfying meals. How does chicken curry sound? You can consume it on the Sirtfood Diet. What about a nice turmeric salmon? That is also a meal that you can enjoy. You can even enjoy blueberry pancakes for breakfast as well.

Sirtfood Diet is the result of extensive studies on a group of proteins called sirtuins, which are regulators of metabolism and which control the ability to burn fat and allow our body to remain in health, acting in many body functions and helping also to live longer and to prevent many pathologies.

The diet was created in 2016 and since then it has been backed up not only by several researches on sirtuin rich foods benefits but also by many epic transformations like the one that saw famous singer Adele losing an impressive amount of 30 kg in just a few months. The same singer, after her reappearance in the newspapers, admitted that the miraculous weight loss was the result of a carefully planned Sirtfood diet.

This diet is a real revolution to keep healthy and maintain results, a real food model capable of making us lose weight without suffering. This is why it has been approved by doctors and nutritionists around the world Let's go in deep and analyze what the Sirtfood Diet exactly is and why it is effective.

Chapter 1. What is the Sirtfood Diet?

The Sirtfood Diet regime takes its name from sirt1, a protein that inhibits fat and positively impacts the metabolism of the fats themselves. Certain foods, in particular, are able to speed up weight loss, allowing to lose up to three and a half pounds a week.

Unlike many other diets, it is not based on fasting, which in many cases is responsible for a feeling of hunger, irritability and loss of muscle mass.

The Sirtfood Diet involves the introduction of a group of very nutrient-rich foods into daily meals named sirtuins that can activate the thinness genes, the same that are activated when you fast, without actually forcing a person to fast for real.

Sirtuins became quite known thanks to research conducted in 2013. In that year it was seen that resveratrol, a substance contained in grapes and red wine, would have the same effects that would be obtained with a calorie restriction. Thanks to this study, it was decided to investigate the topic and find other foods with the same properties.

The scientific reason behind the Sirtfood Diet lies in the fact that sirtuin activators have several health benefits, including building muscles, suppressing appetite, improving memory and controlling blood sugar, cleansing free radicals that accumulate in cells.

Resveratrol is a good example of antioxidant, anti-swelling and vasoprotector while other plant pigments, for their part, have chemical substance that prevents liver damage and antioxidant actions.

When Goggins and Matten got together to study sirtfoods they obviously tested it before releasing it and ultimately designed a diet to maximize sirtfood intake while encouraging mild calorie restrictions.

This is because in their test group of people involved in the first studies of the benefits of this diet, they found that on average, participants who consumed sirtuin-rich foods and restricted their calories between 1000 and 1500kCal for very few days were actually able to see impressive weight loss, even without any increase in exercising or activity.

On average, during that first week, the members lost 7 pounds without doing much else other than changing their diet. Does that sound promising to you?

Even better, these people reported that they were able to gain muscle rather than losing it—something that is practically unheard of in the diet world.

Typically, weight loss comes with muscle loss as well, but these individuals built it. They also reported that they were happier and healthier in general—their mental health and general wellbeing increased as well.

Overall, there are some pretty compelling reasons to start considering the Sirtfood Diet—if you want to lose weight, gain muscle, and be healthier; this is a great way to do this.

Of course it will take some diligence and dedication, but if you can make sure that you commit to this process, you, too, can reap these benefits. You can begin to be a healthier individual, inside and out.

The diet is designed to last three weeks period. At the end of these three weeks, you are encouraged to continue consuming the sirtfoods and drinking green juice. You may also decide to repeat the plan again if you feel the need to.

This Book is structured to guide you through the three weeks of the Sirtfood Diet and offers also a fourth – transition week to give an example of how sirtuin rich foods can be included in an everyday eating plan without effort and with a tasty, pleasant, fulfilling result.

Whether you are vegetarian, vegan, or meat-lover, you will make this diet work for you. All you have to do is follow the guidelines that you will be provided with shortly.

Main Benefits of the Diet

While it is still fully researched and explored, the evidence currently points out that there is a wide range of benefits to the use of sirtuin activation.

The most interesting fact is that those benefits basically derive by including in everyday diet foods that are easy to find and the most people already enjoy consuming, of course in the right proportions and formulations to give us the body structure and health we need.

Appreciating these benefits doesn't require you to implement extreme calorie restrictions for long periods of time, nor does it require grueling exercise regimens (although staying consistently active is a good thing, of course).

Let's go over some of the most common benefits now.

You Will Lose Weight

The most obvious of the benefits is that you will lose weight on this diet. Whether you are exercising or not, there is no way that you would not lose weight when you follow the diet to the letter.

This diet will have you restrict your calories enough so that anyone would lose weight. The average person uses around 2000 calories per day, and this diet will work to have you cut that in half; you will be providing yourself with just 1000 or 1500 calories based on the phase that you are in.

Weight loss is caused by a calorie deficit—it is as simple as that. When you restrict your calories, but you keep your metabolism up, you will find that you will naturally lose weight. This is normal. However, usually, that weight loss is a mix between fat and muscle. As you lose weight and muscle, you would then naturally see your metabolism slow as well. Of course, this means that over time, your weight loss plan is not nearly as effective as it was supposed to be, and as a direct result, you will have to cut calories further to keep that deficit between consumed calories and the calories that your body naturally burns. This means that weight loss eventually slows, or even plateaus if all you do is make use of a weight-loss regimen through cutting calories. You will lose muscle if you are not careful with the weight loss regimen and that will work against you.

However, thanks to the fact that you do not lose muscle mass during the Sirtfood Diet, you do not have to worry about this problem; you simply continue to lose weight because you are able to maintain your metabolism at levels that will keep you continuing to lose weight.

Your Appetite Will Slow

Though your first few days you may find that you are ravenous as your body adjusts to its new normal, over time, you should find this sensation will begin to slow down.

Your body will adjust to the restrictions in calories, and you will be okay with the lower calorie days, especially because the food that you will be eating will include nutrient-dense food that will help your body feel like it is more satisfied.

Veggies and buckwheat are very nutritious foods that are featured heavily in this diet, and you are able to add healthy fats, such as olive oil, to your diet so that you can feel truly satisfied, knowing that ultimately, you have given yourself enough to keep your body going. You will find that you will be able to tolerate the lower amounts of food, and that is a huge plus.

Sirtfoods Have Anti-Aging Effect

Anti-aging is somehow linked to autophagy, which is an intracellular process of repairing or replacing damaged cell parts. This is rejuvenation at an intracellular level. We can't mention autophagy without at least saying something about AMPK, an enzyme very important for cell energy stability. This enzyme helps you boost the energy by activating fatty acid, glucose, and chemical reactions when the cell energy is weak. It represents the body's response when facing an elevated energy demand (e.g., an intense physical exercise).

However, a part of this response is the lysosomal degradation pathway autophagy. Now you are probably wondering what sirtuins have to do with all of these. Well, SIRT1 can activate

AMPK (and the other way around), so it can be considered one of the triggers of autophagy. Autophagy rejuvenates the cell, and this process can happen in all the cells of your body: from the ones of your internal organs to the ones of your skin.

There are a few ways to induce autophagy, and it obviously has a very positive effect on your health and overall lifespan.

Just think of the cell as a car and autophagy is the skilled mechanic capable of fixing or replacing any broken parts in it. Obviously, the cell will have a longer life, and this will impact to your overall life. If your cells are functioning properly, like a Swiss mechanical clock, then you can expect increased longevity.

You can't reverse aging, as there is no such cure for it, and autophagy is not "the fountain of youth." However, this process can significantly slow down aging and its effect. And the best part is that it can be activated by sirtuins, especially SIRT1.

So far, people were not aware of too many ways to trigger autophagy. Some of them were doing it the hard way through intermittent fasting. Others were trying to induce it through an LCHF diet, like the keto diet. Well, now there is an extra way to activate it, and that is through the Sirtfood Diet.

Chapter 2. How the Diet Is Structured

The Sirtfood Diet is made of two different phases and we are going to analyze them below. This Book includes also a third phase to help you go back to a normal sirtuin-rich everyday diet without effort.

Phase 1: The 7 day 'Hyper success Phase'

Phase 1 will take you through a process of hyper-success, where you will take a huge step towards achieving a slimmer, leaner body.

Duration: 7 days.

What to expect

This Phase is famous for being a clinically proven method to lose 7 pounds in 7 days. This is what is experienced by the vast majority of people following Phase 1 guidelines.

Since all people is different, though, it's very important to specify that in this part of the process you just don't rely on the number on the scale. You may find yourself shrinking and finding your clothes less tight or even too big without even see a true difference on the scale. This may depend on several things, your starting point (if you have to lose a few pounds it's more difficult to see immediate results on the scale), how much muscle mass you will build (which will compensate weight loss) among other reasons. These are all perfect measures of big changes in body composition.

Be mindful of other improvements too, such as well-being, energy levels, and how clean the skin appears.

At the local pharmacy, you can get tests of your general cardiovascular and metabolic well-being to see improvements in factors like blood pressure, blood sugar levels, and blood fats like cholesterol and triglycerides.

Remember, weight loss aside, introducing Sirtfoods into your diet is a huge step in making your body fitter and more disease resistant, setting you up for an exceptionally healthy lifetime.

How to follow Phase 1

We already told that Phase 1 is 7 days long. The week is divided in 2 moments: day 1-3 and day 4-7.

Days 1 to 3: These are the only days where a major caloric restriction occurs: 1,000 calories for the whole day. To put this into perspective, an average woman should consume

2,000 calories per to maintain her current weight, but if she wants to lose about 1 pound per week, then the calorie limit drops to 1,500 calories.

To stay within the given parameters for the first three days, the ideal daily menu includes:

- 3 servings of Green juice
- 1 light snack (optional)
- 1 balanced meal

Day 4 to 7: Calories go up 1,500 calories per day. To meet this requirement, the ideal daily menu includes:

- 2 servings of Green juice
- 1 light snack (optional)
- 2 balanced meal

Both the green juices and the meals will include as much sirtfoods as possible, while keeping recipes very tasty and enjoyable.

If you have noticed, the recommended snacks for each day can be taken either in the morning or in the afternoon. Early risers tend to consume their snack in the morning because of the long period between their breakfasts and lunch.

On the other hand, women who have heavier workloads later in the day prefer to consume their snack in the afternoon for an energy boost. Feel free to pick the meal schedule that works for you.

What to Drink

As said, 2 or 3 daily servings of green juices are already included in the Meal Plan but of course they are not the only thing you can drink.

The most important thing is that they are no-calorie drinks: water, black coffee and green tea which are also great to boost the activation of sirtuin in your body.

One thing you ought to be mindful of is that we don't suggest abrupt major improvements to your daily coffee use. Caffeine withdrawal symptoms may make you feel lousy for a few days; likewise, large increases may be unpleasant for those especially sensitive to caffeine effects. Since some researchers have found that adding milk will reduce the absorption of beneficial nutrients that activate sirtuin, we also recommend drinking coffee black without adding milk. The same has been found for green tea, although adding some lemon juice increases its nutrient absorption to activate sirtuin.

If your taste is more for black or herbal teas, do not hesitate to add these too.

Apple/Orange/Pineapple/... juices and soft drinks are forbidden during this Phase. Instead, consider adding a few sliced strawberries or cucumber and mint to still or sparkling water to make your Sirtfood-infused health cocktail, if you want to spice things up.

Refrigerate for a few hours to have a surprisingly cooling alternative to soft drinks and juices.

Remember that this is the period of hyper-success, and while you can be comforted by the fact that it is just for a week, you need to be a careful: we have alcohol for this week, in the form of red wine but only as a cooking ingredient. Though wine belongs to the same category, alcoholic drinks of any kind are not allowed during this phase.

The Sirtfood Green Juice

The green juice is an integral component of the Sirtfood Diet's Step 1 program. All the fixings are prevailing Sirtfoods, and in every liquid, you get a strong cocktail of expected compounds like apigenin, kaempferol, luteolin, quercetin, and EGCG that work together to switch on your sirtuin and encourage fat elimination.

To that, we have added lemon, as it has been shown that its natural acidity prevents, stabilizes and improves the absorption of the sirtuin-activating nutrients. In some recipes, we added a touch of apple and ginger to taste too. You will find a collection of 24 recipes to choose from so that you will never get bored.

Phase 2: Maintenance

By the beginning of week 2, you should be already noticing a radical change in how you feel and most probably in how you look. Feeling however feeling revived and reenergized is as important looking slimmer and increasingly conditioned.

Phase 2 is studied to keep on the right track, losing more weight (we should say fat!) and stabilizing the positive effects the diet has on your body.

Remember that most of the weight that individuals lose is from fat, and that many put on some muscle. So, once again, give the scale the right value and use other tools to understand how things are proceeding: clothes or a meter to measure yourself are good ideas. Probably, people will start complimenting you for the change too. Use the compliments as a booster to keep focused on your journey and get even bigger results.

Remember also that as you keep going, your health is improving and you're creating the roots for a healthy living afterwards.

Duration: 14 days

How to follow Phase 2

The caloric restriction is now very moderate and you shouldn't even notice it. This is because our attention is not on calorie counting.

For the average person, this is not a practical or successful approach over the long term. Instead, we concentrate on healthy servings, very well-balanced meals, and most notably, stocking up on Sirtfoods so that you can start to benefit from their fat-burning and health-promoting effects.

We've also built the meals in the plan to make them satiating, helping you feel full for longer. That, coupled with Sirtfoods natural appetite-regulating powers, means you're not going to spend the next 14 days feeling hungry, but instead happily relaxed, well-fed, and highly well-nourished. Just like in Phase 1, remember to listen and be guided by your appetite. When you prepare meals according to our guidelines you may find that you are easily full before you finish a meal, in that case stop eating will be ok.

The meal plan includes:

- 1 servings of Green juice
- 2 snacks (optional)
- 3 balanced meal

As already said, meals will have to fit around your schedule so arrange them in order to make your life easier. Maybe you are always busy at work or you at the gym or running around with the children. Maybe you prefer to switch a snack with a meal, just have something quick and easy to hold you over to the following meal. Just do it.

Genuine progress goes past total control. It is not sustainable in time: the eating routine must adapt to everyone's living without stress.

During Phase 1 you consumed 1 to 2 meals daily, which gave you heaps of adaptability over when you ate your meals. In Phase 2, as said, meals will be 3. This is why we highly suggest eating breakfast to start the day in the best way possible.

Having a healthy breakfast sets us ready for the day, raising our levels of vitality and focus. Eating earlier keeps our blood sugar and fat levels in check, in terms of our metabolism. A variety of studies point out that breakfast is a positive idea, usually finding that people who eat breakfast are often less likely to be overweight.

Since this is a very important meal, we kept breakfast recipes very quick and simple, so that everyone will be able to eat it, regardless of his/her crazy busy life. You will also be able to prepare some of them in advance, the day before or in batches to freeze or keep handy.

Dedicating at least a few minutes every morning to breakfast, will yield rewards not only for your day but also for your weight and well-being over the longer term. Sirtfoods action to supercharge our energy levels is considerably more powerful on early morning.

What to drink

As in Phase 1, you will keep having green juice every day all through the Phase. This is to keep high your sirtuin levels. Always consider that you can have the daily green juice whenever it's best for you.

You can have it as soon as you get up, 30 minutes before breakfast, as a mid-morning or mid-afternoon snack. In any case, the green juice will help you feel fuller, longer without arriving at lunch or dinner too hungry. Simply go with whatever works for you.

The other drinks will be as usual: water, black coffee, and tea (preferably green tea).

You will also be allowed one glass of wine per day (optional). This is because red wine is rich in sirtuin-initiating polyphenols, particularly resveratrol and piceatannol. One glass is the perfect amount to get the benefits without affecting weight loss due to high caloric consumption.

No other alcoholic beverage is allowed.

Phase 3: Transition to Normal Healthy Eating

Phase 3 will go back to standard caloric intake, while keeping up sirtfood quantities throughout the day.

The Meal plan will include healthy and delicious recipes to show how it's truly easy to have a sirtuin-rich everyday eating. No stress and mouthwatering plates for every meal of the day.

Duration: 1 week

How to follow Phase 3

Simply Cook the suggested recipes. As usual, you can switch lunch and dinner if it's best for you and arrange meals times to fit your needs.

What to drink

We suggest to keep healthy and avoid sugary and alcoholic beverages, limiting them to special occasions. Red wine can be consumed daily in moderate quantities.

Water, coffee, green tea and other no calorie beverages have no particular limitation.

Chapter 3. Is Sirtfood Diet Right for You?

You may be wondering if the Sirtfood Diet is right for you. If you are currently pregnant or breastfeeding, you may want to postpone this diet because of your particular condition.

If you are already following a restricted plan due to some physical condition, remember to talk to your doctor before making any change.

Remember, even if you cannot follow the Meal plan in this book strictly, there is still a great benefit to adding the sirtuin-rich foods to your diet. As we will address shortly, many of the foods rich in sirtuins are highly nutritious and healthy and they should be included in your diet whether you want to follow the Sirtfood Diet or not.

In any other case, you are likely to find that this diet will be perfectly fine for you. Following the main cases in which the sirtfood diet can prove to be most effective.

Obesity

Sirtuins burn fats quickly, and that's what makes this diet a great help for weight loss. When we study all the cases of the successful sirtfood dieters, we can clearly see how well they fought against obesity. Adele is just one example, who has amazed the world with her 30 pounds of weight loss achievement using the sirtfood diet. So, anyone who isn't able to lose some extra pounds for whatever reason, can switch to sirtfood and try a carefully made plan approved by doctors and nutritionists like the one in this book.

Stress

There is one added advantage that higher sirtuin levels can guarantee and that is the reduction in stress and depression. Research is still being conducted on the relationship between sirtfood and stress, but sirtuin is that element that can enable quick brain cell recovery and boosts brain activity by getting rid of all the unwanted metabolic waste. Efficient brain functioning then leads to a reduction in stress. So, this sirtfood diet can also help with stress relief.

Inflammation

What appears to be weight gain or metabolic inactivity is mostly connected to inflammation of both cells and organs in most cases. This inflammation is both the result and cause of several health problems. Sirtfood does not only prevent inflammation at cellular levels but effectively prevents it at the tissue and organ level.

Aging

Aging seems like a threat to all when those wrinkles start appearing on the skin, and the person feels weakened inside out! Sirtuins can play its part in countering the effects of aging. It helps DNA to prolong its life and also aid in the repair process. Sirtuins are also responsible for apoptosis and leads to the formation of new healthy cells. This is the reason that people who are entering into middle age should consider doing the sirtfood diet so that they could effectively fight the possible signs of aging in the years to come.

No workout

Working out is a good way to lose some pounds but non all the people invest the required time and energy to train properly for many reasons. Sirtfood diet can be used by such individuals. Through this diet, they can manage their weight and lose it even while doing only basic physical activities.

Low or Poor Metabolic Activity

Since sirtuins are mainly responsible for better cell metabolism, lower sirtuin levels in the body can hamper the natural cell activities and hinders the metabolism. Poor metabolic activity results in less physical strength, obesity, hormonal imbalance, low enzyme activity, and several other related problems. The sirtfood diet is therefore suggested to boost the metabolic rate in the body and revitalize both body and mind with new levels of energy.

Chapter 4. Full Sirtuin Ingredients List

Sirtuin activating compounds tend to elevate insulin sensitivity and reduce blood sugar level. The main one are:

- **Polyphenols-** Present in turmeric, curcumin. Moderate amount is needed to have a beneficial effect in the body.
- **Resveratrol-** present in blueberries, red grape, raspberries and peanuts. Helps in combating inflammation and improving heart health.
- **Quercetin-** Present in apples, kale, capers, berries, onion, citrus fruits and helps in combating inflammation.
- **Piceatannol-** Popularly used as herbal medicine in Asian countries. It's present in red wine.
- **Oligonol-** Rich in anti-inflammatory properties and often present in lychees.
- **Fisetin-** improves long term memory and present in strawberries.
- **Omega-3-** present in flaxseeds, fish like salmon, catfish, tilapia etc.
- **Melatonin.**

These compounds are found in the 20 main sirtfoods at the base of the Sirtfood Diet.

They are:

Arugula

This green salad leaf (also known as rocket) is very common in the Mediterranean diet. It has a peppery taste useful for digestive and diuretic purposes and nutrients like quercetin and kaempferol capable of activating sirtuins. This combination has very positive effects on the skin as it can moisturize and improve collagen synthesis.

Buckwheat

This crop, amazing for ecological and sustainable farming, is a fruit seed, not a grain. .

Rich in calcium and other important minerals, it is also one of the best sources for rutin, a sirtuin-activator nutrient.

Capers

They are the flower buds of the caper bush, a plant growing abundantly in the Mediterranean region. It is usually handpicked and preserved, and it has some interesting antidiabetic, anti-inflammatory, antimicrobial, antiviral, and immunomodulatory properties. Capers are also rich in sirtuin-activating nutrients, and they are included in some of the recipes for their rich taste.

Celery

This is a plant used for thousands of years, as in ancient Egypt people were already aware of it and its properties. Back then, it was considered a medicinal plant that can be used for detoxing, cleansing, and preventing diseases. Therefore, celery consumption is very good for your gut, kidney, and liver.

Chilies

This veggie should be in your diet whether you like eating spicy food or not. It contains capsaicin, and this substance makes us savor it even more. Consuming chilies is great for activating sirtuins and it speeds up your metabolism. In fact, the spicier the chili is, the more powerful it is when it comes to activating sirtuins. A recent study showed that people eating spicy food three or four times per week have a 14 percent lower death rate compared to people who eat them less than once a week. Thai chilies are very spicy, so they have a maximum sirtuin-activating effect.

Cocoa and Dark Chocolate

Cocoa was considered sacred by the Aztecs and Mayans, and it was a food type reserved only for the warriors or the elite. Although back then, it was mostly used as a drink; you don't have to dilute it with milk or water to reap the full benefits of it. The best way to consume cocoa and get sirtuin-activating flavonols is by eating dark chocolate. Your choice should have at least 85% cocoa solids in order to be considered as sirtfood.

Coffee

This is a drink enjoyed by most adults out there, and it is considered indispensable by most of them. The caffeine acid is a nutrient known to activate sirtuins, so there's more to drinking coffee than a popular and a very pleasant social activity. It is no secret that coffee is very good to give your metabolism and energy levels a boost.

Extra-Virgin Olive Oil

This oil is perhaps the healthiest form of fats you can think of, and it is not missing from any salad in the Mediterranean diet. The health benefits of consuming this oil are countless. It prevents and fights against diabetes, different types of cancer, osteoporosis, and many more. Plus, the extra-virgin olive oil can be associated with increased longevity, as it also has anti-aging effects. This oil has the right nutrients to activate the sirtuin gene in your body.

Garlic

It has a strong antifungal and antibiotic effect and has been successfully used to treat stomach ulcers. Plus, it can be used to remove waste products from your body. It has amazing effects on your blood pressure, blood sugar level, and your heart. Garlic contains allicin, a nutrient capable of triggering sirtuins, but this nutrient can only be valued if the garlic clove is crushed or finely chopped. This is the main way to use garlic in Sirtfood Meal plan included in this book.

Green Tea

This sirtuin-filled beverage is actually a popular choice for health buffs, making it the world's most consumed beverage after water. It is known to help boost weight loss, prevent Alzheimer's disease, reduce cholesterol build-up, and combat heart diseases. Some of the essential vitamins and minerals it contains are folate, vitamin b, magnesium and other antioxidants. It also contains EGCG (epigallocatechin), which is known to be a very powerful sirtuin activator.

Kale

This is a popular "superfood" since it is filled with antioxidants (beta-carotene, kaempferol, quercetin and more). In fact, this veggie has one of the highest oxygen radical absorbance capacity or orac rating; it is known to be nutrient-dense – it has omega 3 fatty acids, vitamins a, k, C and b6, it also has calcium, potassium, magnesium and more. It can also lower cholesterol levels, has anti-cancer effects and can help you lose weight.

Medjool Dates

If you have the chance to go to any country of the Middle East or the Arabian Peninsula, you will find that dates are a very common snack. Dehydrated, covered in chocolate, or a fresher form, dates are perhaps the most common snack you can find over there.

Now you are probably wondering if it has any health benefits, especially if you find out that Medjool dates have around 66 percent sugar. But sugar in this form is a lot less harmful than processed or refined sugar, which doesn't have any sirtuin-activating properties and can be easily linked to weight gain (even obesity), heart disease, and diabetes.

Parsley

Parsley leaves are extremely frequent in the recipes of the book; they are an easy way to add sirtfoods to your diet. Just chop them and toss them in your meal, with their refreshing and vibrant taste, they will complete it and make it tasty.

This sirtuin food has vitamins A, C and K (richest herbal source for vitamin K) and contains volatile oil and flavonoid. It is also said to help promote osteotropic activity in our bones. It is a great source of apigenin, which is a sirtuin-activating nutrient. This nutrient can rarely be found in such quantities in other food and it can help you relax and easily fall asleep.

Red Endive

The recently found plant is growing all over the world. It plays a major role in a sirtfood diet because of its high concentration of luteolin, a sirtuin-activating nutrient.

A great way to raise the quantity of luteolin in your diet is to add red endive to your salad. Naturally, pour some extra-virgin olive oil to make it more sirtuin-activating. Endives can come in different colors. It would be great if you can find them red (as these are the best), but you can settle for yellow ones as well.

Red Onions

Aside from adding flavor to our dishes, onion is actually a popular component for different home remedies. It is known to heal infection, reduce inflammation and regulates sugar. In addition, it also has high polyphenol content, contains volatile oil and other organic sulfur compounds. It has plenty of antioxidants, and it is known to fight against inflammation, heart diseases, and diabetes. It is a great source for quercetin, an amazing sirtuin-activating nutrient that is believed to enhance sports performance.

Red Wine

The Mediterranean diet encourages the consumption of red wine, and there are plenty of reasons why you should consider the moderate consumption of it. We are not going to talk about the effects it has over your blood, blood sugar level, and so on. Not even about how moderate consumption can decrease the death rates by heart disease. Red wines like Merlot, Cabernet Sauvignon, or Pinot Noir have an incredible concentration of polyphenol to activate your sirtuins.

Soy

It soy contains formononetin and daidzein, two great sirtuin-activating nutrients. In the Meal plan included in this book, it has been added in two different forms: tofu (the vegan protein boost), and miso (a Japanese fermented paste with an intense umami flavor), but you can experiment its many forms in your everyday meals after completing the 4-weeks plan.

Strawberries

Of all the fruits out there, strawberries are among the ones with the most health benefits. For example, they have a very high concentration of fisetin, a nutrient that can activate sirtuins.

The consumption of this fruit can lower the insulin demand, basically turning the food into a sustainable energy releaser. There is research claiming that eating strawberries has similar effects on drug therapy for a person who has diabetes.

Turmeric

Curcumin, a substance found in turmeric, has potent anti-inflammatory effects. Aside from being a strong antioxidant, it is also known for its anti-inflammatory effects. It is also known to help with liver problems, arthritis, heartburn, kidney problems, and even depression. To boost curcumin absorption, cook it in liquid, add some fat and black pepper. This is how it has been frequently added to the recipes in this Book.

Walnuts

Without any doubt, walnuts are the best nuts when it comes to health. They have a high concentration of good fats and a moderate consumption – they are very caloric - is associated with lowering the risk of diabetes, preventing cardiovascular diseases, and lowering body weight. Walnuts are also known for their anti-aging effects and their nutrients are known to activate sirtuins.

Besides the 20 main foods shown above, there are many other sirtfoods you can include in your meals, this will help you having a very colorful and varied diet which will aid fat burning and muscle gain thanks to sirtuin activation.

- Apples
- Artichokes
- Asparagus
- Blackberries
- Blackcurrants
- Blueberries
- Broad beans
- Broccoli
- Chestnuts
- Chia seeds
- Chickpeas
- Chicory
- Chili peppers
- Chives
- Corn
- Cranberries
- Dill
- Endive lettuce
- Ginger
- Goji berries
- Green beans
- Mint
- Oregano
- Pak choi
- Peanuts
- Pistachios
- Plums
- Quinoa
- Raspberries
- Red Grapes
- Sage
- Shallots
- Spinach
- Sunflower seeds
- Watercress
- White Onions

Chapter 5. Meal Prepping Suggestions

In this Book, the Meal plan provided includes many different recipes to let you enjoy variety as much as possible. As you know, after week 4 you transition to normal, healthy eating and you may need to experiment less because you already have many recipes you like. This is when Meal prepping will come handy.

Meal prepping is the activity to cook and pack advance many individual servings of weekly meals and snacks having them fully cooked and boxed. Meal prepping can be done one or two days each week, depending on your individual needs and schedule. The same meal will be divided and boxed for several meals, frozen (if needed) and be ready to heat-and-eat, like a casserole, or eat cold, like a salad. But the benefits of meal prepping go a lot further than just convenience.

Meal prep dos and don'ts

Developing smart meal prepping habits is part of the learning process. Here are some meal prep dos and don'ts worth keeping in mind as you get started:

✔DO Select one or two days to meal prep. Sundays work best for many folks, but another day during the week might work better for you. For example, if you work over the weekend, then a day off during the week is probably a better day for you to meal prep. You can also choose two days each week to prep food.

✔DO flag healthy recipes you love. After trying healthy recipes, keep the ones you love in a folder or mark them in this book or in other cookbooks you already have that you may want to use as inspiration. In this way, when going back to normal healthy eating you will have plenty of ideas to choose from.

✔DO When deciding which recipes to swap into your meal prep schedule, keep variety in mind when it comes to protein, whole grains, and veggies. Nutritionally, this will allow you to take in a wider range of nutrients. If one meal for the week is fish with asparagus, you'll probably want to select a chicken, beef, pork, or vegetarian recipe with a different vegetable to rotate with during the week. At the same time, try to keep some of the ingredients between recipes the same, which can help decrease food costs and help use up an ingredient. For example, if you have a meal for breakfast; plan to use up the remaining ingredients as a fixing for one of the other meals like lunch or dinner meals.

✔DO go at your own pace. You can successfully meal prep with three recipes or six recipes. You don't need to prepare 10 or more recipes for the week. Start slowly and build your way up.

✔ DO To make the most of your time and money, after selecting your recipes, go through the ingredients and check if you have them. List the ingredients you need to purchase according to the flow of your market. For example, if you shop at a traditional supermarket, produce is usually the first place you'll find yourself. Categorize your shopping list in this order: fruits, vegetables and herbs, milk and dairy, proteins (like meat, chicken, and fish), packaged goods, and frozen items. Note how much you need of each ingredient to avoid buying too much.

✔ DO work with your schedule. Some weeks you'll be able to prepare more recipes than other weeks. Does whatever work for you and your schedule.

✔ DO freeze extras. Some weeks you will have a few extra meals. Freezer-friendly meals can be frozen and kept for up to a few months, as noted in the recipes.

✔ DO make cleanup easy. You'll have many vegetable scraps, eggshells, and empty containers to toss, so keep your recycling, compost bin, and trash nearby for easy cleanup.

✘ DON 'T wait too long. Plan ahead for best results. Meal prepping is about scheduling your time in advance, so you can get to the market and buy the ingredients you need, then spend the necessary time at home preparing them.

✘ DON'T divide meals later. The last step of meal prepping is to divide recipes into individual portions and pack them into containers. Don't skip this step or divide meals right before digging into one. Dividing meals up front helps maintain good portion control, prevents last-minute scrambling to divide meals, and ensures your meals will last through the week.

✘ DON'T over prep. The last thing you want to do is prep meals that will go uneaten, unless of course you can freeze them. To get into the meal prepping jive, start slow and get to know your meal prepping needs.

Chapter 6. Why aren't you losing weight?

Let's clarify a common doubt. You feel that you are already eating some sirtfoods you read about in this book. So why didn't you lose weight already? Here's why.

Hitting Your Quota

Most people just don't eat nearly enough Sirtfoods to enjoy a strong fat-burning and fitness-boosting influence. The average intake of five basic sirtuin-activating compounds (quercetin, luteolin, myricetin, kaempferol, and apigenin) in the US diet has been found to be a miserable 13mg a day.

To give you an idea, Japanese daily consumption is more than 5 times greater and as already told Japanese people are among the best consumers in the world of sirtuin-rich foods.

This book is studied to allow you to improve your intake many times (in some cases up to 50 times) in a way that fits your busy schedule. You can indeed efficiently and cheaply reach the level of consumption needed to gain all of the benefits.

The Power of Synergy

The smartest way to guarantee our body the correct intake of nutrients is by eating a vast variety of whole food (organic, where possible).

Along with main nutrients we all know, whole foods contain dozens of less known compounds the work together in synergy to increase our wellbeing.

It has been proven by several studies that single nutrient supplementation does not give the same permanent effect in time than the same component that has been included in the diet in form of whole food.

Take, for example, the basic component resveratrol which activates sirtuin. This could be consumed in supplementary form; but its bioavailability (how much the person can actually absorb it) is at least 6 times higher if got through red wine.

This is because red wine includes not just resveratrol but also a complete variety of sirtuin-activating polyphenols like myricetin, piceatannol, quercetin and epicatechin that work with each other to offer positive effects,.

Another example is curcumin, which is the main sirtuin-activating ingredient in turmeric. It has been proven that turmeric has much stronger PPAR action to enhance fat burning and is much more capable of suppressing cancer and decreasing blood glucose levels than isolated curcumin.

This is why, unlike many other diets, supplements are not recommended: supplementing a single nutrient is nowhere near as successful as eating it.

Combining multiple Sirtfoods is what really makes this book and its 4-weeks Meal plan special. For example, introducing quercetin-rich Sirtfoods boosts the benefits of resveratrol contained in other foods. Resveratrol is very effective in promoting deterioration of mature fat cells, while quercetin is active in preventing new fat tissue from developing.

Foods that are high in sirtuin enhancer apigenin boost the quercetin intake from diet and increase its function.

Quercetin has been proven to work in synergy with epigallocatechin gallate (EGCG). And EGCG's work with curcumin has been seen to be complementary. So, not only are individual whole products more effective than single nutrient supplements, but combining several sirtuin-rich foods give even more benefits thanks to the synergy between the compounds.

Juicing and Food: Get the Best of Both Worlds

As explained Sirtfood Diet combines freshly made juices and whole food products. For some people that may sound counterintuitive, based on the fact that the fiber is lost while ingredients are juiced. Yet this is just what we need, especially from leafy green vegetables.

This is because they contain not only sirtuin-activating polyphenols but also non-extractable polyphenols (or NEPPs) bound to the fibrous portion of the food. NEPPs cannot be processed by the body and are simply eliminated as waste.

So, by juicing them and eliminating the low-nutrient material, we obtain an amazingly concentrated dose of sirtuin-activating polyphenols, with no trace of the bad components which undermine our health.

There is yet another benefit of cutting the fibers, too. The type of fiber in green leafy vegetables contain is called non - soluble fiber and it has a gastrointestinal scrubbing action. When we consume too much of it, we disrupt digestive lining possibly aggravating or even inducing IBS (irritable bowel syndrome) and obstructing nutrient intake.

Without fiber, the digestion of ingredients (like matcha tea, for example) has been proven much more successful when combined to a green juice and this is true for many essential nutrients, like magnesium and folic acid.

Chapter 7. Tips to Get Max Results

Here some common tips from Nutritionists all around the world to help you get the most from Sirtfood Diet.

Drink water

Thirst can be confused with food or hunger cravings. In case you're feeling that sudden urge to get a particular food, try drinking a massive glass of water and then wait for a couple of minutes. You might discover that the craving disappears as your body was actually only thirsty.

Moreover, drinking a lot of water might have many health benefits, for example: water before meals can lower hunger and help with weight reduction.

Eat Early

It is proven that having the last meal by 7 p.m. is best for several reasons. First of all, it' much better to benefit from Sirtfoods natural satiating power starting early in the morning. Having food that will leave you feeling full, happy, and energetic as you go about your day is more effective than passing the whole day feeling hungry and eat most of your food late, not having enough time to completely digest it before going to bed, impacting on your sleep.

Eat the right amount of protein

Sirtfood foods are proven to work best with the correct amount of protein per meal. In particular, specific protein leucine helps SIRT1 to enhance fat loss and boost blood sugar regulation.

Leucine has also another role which is inducing anabolism (building things) in our cells, especially in muscles. Anabolism is an activity which requires a great deal of energy and ensures that our energy producers (called mitochondria) have to work extra hours. Sirtfood support this activity, increasing the growth of more mitochondria, boosting their efficiency, and making them burn fat as fuel. As you can see there is a synergic action between sirtuins and proteins like leucine and this synergy eventually allows you to lose fat to support muscle development and better safety.

Plan meals

If possible, attempt to organize your diet daily or weekly. This Book gives you an example of what a month of good planning could be offering a lot of solutions for your meals.

By understanding what you are going to consume, you get rid of the variable of spontaneity and doubt that could result in cravings or wrong choices.

Avoid getting too hungry

Hunger is among the primary reasons why people experience cravings. To avoid becoming too hungry, the best things to do are eating regularly and have healthy snacks at hand. By being ready, and preventing too many hours of fasting, you will protect yourself against the cravings.

Fight stress

Stress may cause cravings for food and influence eating behaviors. Unfortunately, people enduring stressful situations for too long are demonstrated to eat more calories and experience more significant cravings compared to non-stressed people.

Try to minimize stress in your environment by addressing it early, meditating and generally, slowing down.

Get enough sleep

Your appetite is mainly affected by hormones that change during your daytime. Studies support this, revealing that sleep-deprived men and women are up to 55 percent more likely to gain weight, in comparison to folks who have enough sleep.

Sleep deprivation might interrupt ordinary changes in desire hormones, resulting in cravings and inadequate appetite control. Put your phone down at least 2 hours before going to bed to avoid disrupting your sleep.

Eat proper meals

Scarcity of essential nutrients may cause cravings. It is critical to eat proper healthy foods most of the times so that the body is guaranteed the nutrients it needs and does not cause hard to manage cravings.

Do not go to the grocery if you are starving

Grocery stores are most likely the hardest places to be whenever you're hungry. Have a light snack and a big glass of water before going, prepare a complete shopping list including all the items you need and buy just those. In this way you won't have to think much about other foods and will spend less in time in a place that may cause you to fall off the wagon.

Distance yourself in the craving

When you're feeling that craving, make an effort to distance yourself from it. For example, you'll be able to have a brisk walk or perhaps a shower to alter the mind onto something different. A significant change in environment and thought might help block the craving.

Exercise mindful eating

Mindful eating is all about practicing mindfulness, a kind of meditation, even in regard to eating and foods. Mindful eating educates to distinguish between cravings and actual hunger. It makes it possible to select your answer to both of them, rather than acting on it thoughtlessly or impulsively. It instructs to go in deep in the comprehension of the meal plan, feelings, appetite and cravings, and bodily senses.

Chapter 8. 4-Weeks Meal Plan

This is without any doubt the most important section of the Book, where you will be able to learn about your new healthy way of eating in the next 4 weeks.

Here you will fully understand what following a Sirtfood Diet means and find out how easy it is to reach your goals while making significant and lifetime changes that will guarantee weight loss results that last and an improved health condition. Just follow the instructions and the month will fly by without even noticing it.

But before starting, let's talk about pantry basics.

Pantry basics

The following ingredients are probably already in your pantry.

If not, add them <u>once</u> to have them handy during the next 4 weeks (but most of them will last much longer, even months).

Cooking basics:

Baking powder, Basmati rice Bread Crumbs, Brown Rice, Capers, Cocoa powder, Canned Tomatoes, Coconut Oil, Cooking Spray, Extra Virgin Olive Oil, Flour, Honey, Oats, Red wine, Sesame oil, Stock cubes, Tomato sauce.

Dressings:

Balsamic Vinegar, Mustard, Salt, Soy Sauce, Tamari.

Herbs and Spices:

Bay, Basil, Chili, Cinnamon, Cumin, Curry, Dill, Garam Masala, Garlic, Ginger, Marjoram, Nutmeg, Oregano, Paprika, Pepper, Rosemary, Sage, Thyme, Turmeric, Vanilla Extract.

Nuts and Seeds:

Almonds, Pumpkin seeds, Sesame seeds, Walnuts.

Week 1 – Phase 1: The 7 day 'Hyper success Phase' quick recap

This week is divided in two moments:
Day 1-3 with 3 juices a day, 1 optional snack and a full meal.
Day 4-7 with 2 juices a day, 2 optional snacks and a full meal.

Week 1 – Phase 1 – Shopping List

Artichokes	Chicken Wings	Red Peppers
Arugula	Chicory	Salmon
Avocado	Coconut cream	Shrimps
Baby Spinach	Dates	Smoked Salmon
Bird's eye chili	Goat Cheese	Spinach
Broccoli	Kale	Sweet potatoes
Buckwheat	Lettuce	Tomatoes
Buckwheat flour	Leeks	Tuna Steak
Carrots	Lemons	Turkey Breast
Celeriac	Orange	Turnips
Celery	Parmesan	Yellow Peppers
Chicken Breast	Parsley	
Chicken Thighs	Red Onions	

<u>Important:</u> The Plan lets you choose your favorite Sirtfood Green Juices Recipes each week, remember to include the related ingredients in this list accordingly.

Week 1 – Phase 1 – Meal Plan

DAY	BREAKFAST	SNACK	LUNCH	SNACK	DINNER
MON	Sirtfood Green Juice (page 50)	2 squares of dark chocolate	Sirtfood Green Juice (page 50)	Sirtfood Green Juice (page 50)	Sweet Potato and Salmon Patties Raw Artichoke Salad (pages 113/114)
TUE	Sirtfood Green Juice (page 50)	2 squares of dark chocolate	Sirtfood Green Juice (page 50)	Sirtfood Green Juice (page 50)	Lemon Paprika Chicken with Vegetables (page 115)
WED	Sirtfood Green Juice (page 50)	2 squares of dark chocolate	Sirtfood Green Juice (page 50)	Sirtfood Green Juice (page 50)	Tomato Soup with Meatballs (page 116)
THU	Sirtfood Green Juice (page 50)	Sirtfood Green Juice (page 50)	Chicken with Kale and Chili Salsa (page 117)	2 squares of dark chocolate	Seared Tuna in Soy Sauce and Black Pepper (page118)
FRI	Sirtfood Green Juice (page 50)	Sirtfood Green Juice (page 50)	Sirt Salmon Salad (page 50)	2 squares of dark chocolate	Green Veggies Curry (page 120)
SAT	Sirtfood Green Juice (page 50)	Sirtfood Green Juice (page 50)	Shrimp Tomato Stew (page 121)	2 squares of dark chocolate	Turkey Breast with Peppers (page 122)
SUN	Sirtfood Green Juice (page 50)	Sirtfood Green Juice (page 50)	Goat Cheese Salad with Cranberries and Walnut (page 123)	2 squares of dark chocolate	Spicy Chicken Stew (page 124)

Week 2 and 3 – Phase 2: 'Maintenance Phase' Quick Recap

This week is divided in two moments:
Week 2 with 1 juice a day, 2 optional snacks and 2 full meals.
Week 3 with 1 juice a day, 2 optional snacks and 2 full meals.

Week 2 – Phase 2 – Shopping List

Almond Milk, unsweetened	Chocolate, 85%	Parmesan
Arugula	Coconut milk, full fat	Parsley
Asparagus	Cucumber	Parsnip
Avocado	Eggs	Red Onions
Baby Spinach	Greek yoghurt	Red Peppers
Banana	Kale	Salmon fillets
Bird's eye chili	Lean Mince	Scallions
Blueberries	Lettuce	Shrimps
Broccoli	Lemons	Sirloin
Buckwheat, puffed	Lentils, canned	Strawberries
Carrots	Lime	Tomatoes
Cauliflower	Milk, skimmed	Trout fillets
Celeriac	Mixed Berries, frozen	Turkey Breast
Celery	Mozzarella	Turnips
Cherry tomatoes	Mushrooms	Yellow Peppers
Chicken Wings	Oats	
Chicory	Orange	

<u>Important:</u> The Plan lets you choose your favorite Sirtfood Green Juices Recipes each week, remember to include the related ingredients in this list accordingly.

Week 2 – Phase 2 – Meal Plan

DAY	BREAKFAST	SNACK	LUNCH	SNACK	DINNER
MON	Fluffy Blueberry Pancakes (page125)	Sirtfood Green Juice (page 50)	Caprese Skewers (page 126)	2 squares of dark chocolate	Baked Salmon with Stir Fried Vegetables (page 127)
TUE	Kale and Mushroom Frittata (page 128)	Sirtfood Green Juice (page 50)	Trout with Roasted Vegetables (page 129)	Banana Strawberry Smoothie (page 130)	Mince Stuffed Peppers (page 131)
WED	Vanilla Parfait with Berries (page 132)	Sirtfood Green Juice (page 50)	Arugula Salad with Turkey and Italian Dressing (page 133)	2 squares of dark chocolate	Creamy Mushroom Soup with Chicken (page 134)
THU	Super Easy Scrambled Eggs and Cherry Tomatoes (page 135)	Sirtfood Green Juice (page 50)	Lemon Ginger Shrimp Salad (page 136)	Blueberry Smoothie (page 137)	Lemon Chicken Skewers with Peppers (page 137)
FRI	Overnight Oats with Strawberries and Chocolate (page 138)	Sirtfood Green Juice (page 50)	Spicy Salmon with Turmeric and Lentils (page 139)	2 squares of dark chocolate	Chicken and Broccoli Creamy Casserole (page 140)
SAT	Sautéed Mushrooms and Poached Eggs (page 141)	Sirtfood Green Juice (page 50)	Asian Beef Salad (page 141)	Chocolate Mousse (page 142)	Creamy Turkey and Asparagus (page 143)
SUN	Banana Vanilla Pancake (page 144)	Sirtfood Green Juice (page 50)	Shredded Chicken Bowl (page 145)	2 squares of dark chocolate	Indian Vegetarian Meatballs (page 146)

Week 3 – Phase 2 – Shopping List

Almond Milk, unsweetened
Artichokes
Arugula
Avocado
Banana
Bird's eye chili
Blueberries
Brussels Sprouts
Buckwheat
Carrots
Celery
Cheddar
Cherry tomatoes
Chicken Breast
Chickpeas, canned
Cilantro

Eggplants
Eggs
Feta cheese
Greek yoghurt
Kale
Lettuce
Lemons
Milk, skimmed
Mint
Mixed Berries, frozen
Miso Paste
Mozzarella
Mushrooms
Oats
Orange
Parmesan

Parsley
Plain Yoghurt
Red Onions
Ricotta cheese
Salmon fillets
Scallions
Sirloin
Spinach
Sweet potatoes
Tomato paste
Tomatoes
Tortillas, wholegrain
Tuna Steak
Turkey Bacon
Turkey Breast

Important: The Plan lets you choose your favorite Sirtfood Green Juices Recipes each week, remember to include the related ingredients in this list accordingly.

Week 3 – Phase 2 – Meal Plan

DAY	BREAKFAST	SNACK	LUNCH	SNACK	DINNER
MON	Blueberry and Walnut Bake (page 147)	Sirtfood Green Juice (page 50)	Shrimp Tomato Stew (page 121)	Buckwheat Granola (page 148)	Turkey Bacon Fajitas (page 149)
TUE	Brussels Sprouts Egg Skillet (page 150)	Sirtfood Green Juice (page 50)	Orange Cumin Sirloin Simple Arugula Salad (pages 151/152)	2 squares of dark chocolate	Garlic Salmon with Brussel Sprouts and Rice (page 153)
WED	Banana Vanilla Pancake (page 144)	Sirtfood Green Juice (page 50)	Indian Vegetarian Meatballs (page 146)	Blueberry Smoothie (page 137)	Sesame Glazed Chicken with Ginger and Chili Stir-Fried Greens (page 154)
THU	Super Easy Scrambled Eggs and Cherry Tomatoes (page 135)	Sirtfood Green Juice (page 50)	Brussels Sprouts and Ricotta Salad (page 155)	2 squares of dark chocolate	Sesame Tuna with Artichoke Hearts (page 156)
FRI	Fluffy Blueberry Pancakes (page125)	Sirtfood Green Juice (page 50)	Baked Salmon with Stir Fried Vegetables (page 127)	Chocolate Mousse (page 142)	Spicy Stew with Potatoes and Spinach (page 157)
SAT	Sautéed Mushrooms and Poached Eggs (page 141)	Sirtfood Green Juice (page 50)	Roasted Butternut and Chickpeas Salad (page 158)	2 squares of dark chocolate	Eggplant Pizza Towers (page 159)
SUN	Vanilla Parfait with Berries (page 132)	Sirtfood Green Juice (page 50)	Arugula Salad with Turkey and Italian Dressing (page 133)	Mango Mousse with Chocolate Chips (page 160)	Greek Frittata with Garlic Grilled Eggplant (page 161)

Week 4 – Phase 3: Transition Quick Recap

After completing successfully Phase 1 and 2, Phase 3 will allow you to transition to normal healthy eating that keep including a variety of Sirtfoods in daily meals.

Week 4: 1 juice a day, 2 snacks and 3 full meals.

Week 4 – Transition – Shopping List

Almond Milk, unsweetened	Chicken Breast	Parmesan
Almond Flour	Chicken Mince	Parsley
Arugula	Chickpeas, canned	Peanut Butter
Avocado	Chicory	Potatoes
Baby potatoes	Coconut, shredded	Red Onions
Baby Spinach	Dates	Red Peppers
Banana	Eggs	Ricotta cheese
Blueberries	Lamb, shoulder	Shrimps
Broccoli	Lean Mince	Spinach
Brussels Sprouts	Lettuce	Strawberries
Buns, whole wheat	Lentils, canned	Sweet potatoes
Butternut Squash	Mozzarella	Tomatoes
Buckwheat	Mushrooms	Tuna Steak
Cheddar	Oats	Wine

<u>Important:</u> The Plan lets you choose your favorite Sirtfood Green Juices Recipes each week, remember to include the related ingredients in this list accordingly.

Week 4 – Phase 3 – Meal Plan

DAY	BREAKFAST	SNACK	LUNCH	SNACK	DINNER
MON	Brussels Sprouts Egg Skillet (page 150)	Chocolate Mousse (page 142)	Creamy Turkey and Asparagus (page 143)	Sirtfood Green Juice (page 50)	Spicy Indian Dahl with Basmati Rice (page 162)
TUE	Vanilla Parfait with Berries (page 132)	Sirtfood Green Juice (page 50)	Lemony Chicken Burgers (page 163)	Walnut Energy Bar (page 164)	Sesame Tuna with Artichoke Hearts Baked Sweet Potato (page 156/165)
WED	Blueberry and Walnut Bake (page 147)	Mango Mousse with Chocolate Chips (page 160)	Shredded Chicken Bowl (page 145)	Sirtfood Green Juice (page 50)	Creamy Broccoli and Potato Soup (page 166)
THU	Chickpea Fritters (page 167)	Sirtfood Green Juice (page 50)	Lemon Tuna Steaks with Baby Potatoes (page 168)	Chocolate Mousse (page 142)	Lamb, Butternut Squash and Date Tagine (page 169)
FRI	Fluffy Blueberry Pancakes (page125)	2 squares of dark chocolate	Lemon Ginger Shrimp Salad (page 136)	Sirtfood Green Juice (page 50)	Mince Stuffed Peppers (page 131)
SAT	Overnight Oats with Strawberries and Chocolate (page 138)	Sirtfood Green Juice (page 50)	Chicken and Broccoli Creamy Casserole Baked Sweet Potato(page 140/165)	Buckwheat Granola (page 148) ½ cup plain yoghurt	Spinach Quiche (page 170)
SUN	Banana Vanilla Pancake (page 144)	Sirtfood Green Juice (page 50)	Brussels Sprouts and Ricotta Salad (page 155)	Energy Cocoa Balls (page 171)	Mexican Chicken Casserole (page 172)

Recipes

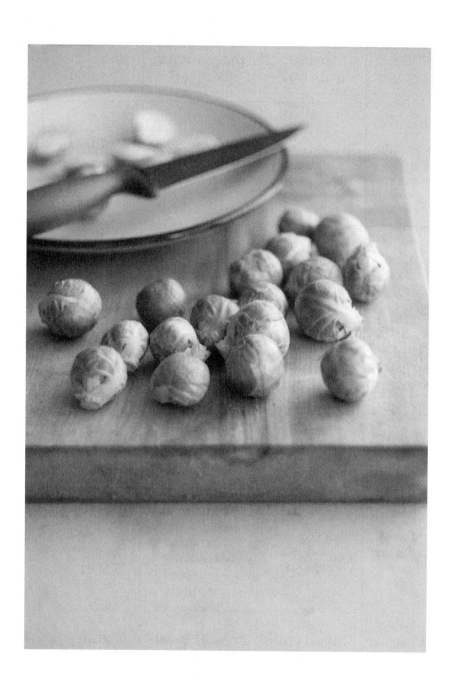

Chapter 9. Sirtfood Green Juice Collection

Below you can find a collection of 24 different recipes to choose from for your daily Green Juices. Simply go for your favorite one or try them all! It's up to you.

1 grapefruit ½ lemon ½ spirulina sparkling water	2 apples ¼ white cabbage ½ fennel 3 mint leaves	2 apples 1 cucumber 1-inch ginger 3 mint leaves
2 apples ¼ lettuce ½ lemon ½ tsp matcha tea	2 apples 2 kale leaves 1 stick celery 1/3 cucumber ½ beetroot	1 cucumber 2 apples 1-inch ginger 2 mint leaves
1 cucumber 2 pears ½ lemon handful lovage	1 cucumber 3 tomatoes handful parsley ½ lemon	1 cucumber 1 apple 1 stick celery ½ lemon
1 handful parsley ½ apple 4 broccoli florets ½ grapefruit	8 broccoli florets handful parsley 3 apples	8 broccoli florets 2 sticks celery 2 pears
2 cups spinach 2 stick celery 2 oranges	8 broccoli florets 2 grapefruit ½ tsp matcha tea	2 kale leaves 2 apples ½ cucumber
handful parsley ¼ white cabbage ½ cucumber ½ melon	½ lettuce 2 apples ½ lemon ½ cup spinach	handful parsley 1 lemon 5 tomatoes

1 cup spinach 2 mint leaves ½ pineapple	2 grapefruits ¼ red cabbage ½ tsp matcha tea	2 grapefruits ½ fennel 1 apple 3 mint leaves
1 grapefruit ½ cucumber 1 celery 2 mint leaves	1 orange 1 carrot 1 cucumber 1 stick celery	1 orange 1 carrot 1 stick celery 1-inch ginger

Preparation Time: 5 minutes

Number of Servings: 2

Directions:

Choose one of the recipes in the table above.

Add all ingredients into a juicer and extract the juice according to the manufacturer's method.

In case you don't have one, add all the ingredients in a blender and pulse until well combined.

Filter the juice through a fine mesh strainer and transfer into two glasses.

Serve immediately.

Avg. Nutrition Facts: Calories 32kcal, Fat 0.5 g, Carbohydrate 6.5 g, Protein 1 g

Chapter 10.   Week 1 Recipes

Sweet Potato and Salmon Patties

Preparation time: 10 minutes

Cooking time: 30 minutes

Servings: 2

Ingredients:

3 tbsp. Buckwheat flour

8oz wild salmon, cooked or tinned

8oz sweet potato cooked and mashed

1 tbs. dill

1 head red endive

1 tbsp. extra virgin olive oil

1 tbsp. balsamic vinegar

Directions:

Preheat the oven up to 325°F.

Mix the sweet potato, salmon, dill, salt and pepper together. Take a small handful of mixture and shape it into a ball. Flatten into a shape of burger then dip into the flour on each side. Place it on a lined baking tray. Repeat until the blend is used up.

Bake only turning once for 20 minutes. Serve with a salad made with finely sliced red endive seasoned with vinaigrette made with olive oil, salt, pepper and vinegar.

Nutrition Facts: Calories: 316 kcal, Fat: 6.3g, Carbohydrate: 18.3g, Protein: 19.2g

Raw Artichoke Salad

Preparation time: 5 minutes

Cooking time: 15 minutes

Servings: 2

Ingredients:

2 Roman artichokes

1 lemon, juice

1 tsp. extra virgin olive oil

Salt and pepper

Directions:

Wash and peel the artichokes by removing all the hardest leaves. Cut them in two and gently remove the hair inside the artichoke.

Cut them very finely (using a mandolin if you have one)

Put them in water and lemon so that they do not turn brown.

When ready to serve, drain the artichokes, mix them with olive oil, a few drops of lemon, salt and pepper and put them on a serving plate.

Nutrition Facts: Calories: 100 Fat: 10.9g Protein: 13.3g Carbohydrate: 3.4g

Lemon Paprika Chicken with Vegetables

Preparation time: 10 minutes

Cooking time: 45 minutes

Servings: 2

Ingredients:

2 carrots, chopped

2 bay leaves

2 tbsp. red wine

Juice of 1 lemon

½ celeriac, peeled and chopped

3 turnips, peeled and chopped

8 oz. of chicken wings

3 tbsp. extra virgin olive oil

2 tbsp. paprika

2 cups stock

Sprigs of rosemary and thyme

2 cups kale, chopped

Directions:

Heat the oil with a tight fitting lid inside a large saucepan. Add the carrots, paprika, celeriac, turnips and chicken wings to the saucepan and cook for a few minutes. Add the wine, mix and let it evaporate.

Stir in the pan the stock, spices, salt, pepper and lemon juice and bring to the boil.

Turn the heat down, cover it with a lid and gently simmer for 40 minutes.

Add the kale and cook until the kale and the chicken are both cooked for a few more minutes.

Nutrition Facts: Calories 154.0 Total Fat 2.2 g Carbohydrate: 32.1 Protein 21.4

Tomato Soup with Meatballs

Preparation time: 15 minutes

Cooking time: 30 minutes

Servings: 2

Ingredients:

8 oz. lean mince

1 egg

1 tbsp. parmesan

1 tbsp. breadcrumbs

2 tsp. of extra virgin olive oil

1 red onion finely chopped

1 yellow pepper, chopped

1 red pepper, chopped

1 can tomatoes or 3 ripe large tomatoes

2 cups stock

1 clove of garlic, crushed

1 chili, finely sliced

4 oz. buckwheat

salt and pepper to taste

Directions:

Put mince, egg, breadcrumbs, parmesan, salt and pepper in a bowl and mix well, then create small meatballs.

Heat a pan, add oil and gently sauté onion and garlic until transparent.

Add the meatballs and cook another 5 minutes.

Add peppers and chili and let flavors mix together, then add the tomatoes (canned or roughly chopped if fresh), add the broth and let it simmer for 20-25 minutes.

While the soup cooks, boil buckwheat for 25 minutes, drain it and add it to the soup right before serving it.

Nutrition Facts: Calories: 348, Fat: 7.6g, Carbohydrate: 28.4g, Protein: 23.2g

Chicken with Kale and Chili Salsa

Preparation time: 5 minutes

Cooking time: 40 minutes

Servings: 3

Ingredients:

3 oz. buckwheat

1 tsp. fresh ginger

½ lemon, juiced

1 tsp. turmeric

2 cups kale, chopped

1 oz. onion, sliced

8 oz. chicken breast

2tsp. extra virgin olive oil

1 tomato

1 handful parsley

1 bird's eye chili, chopped

1tsp. paprika

Directions:

Finely chop the tomato, mix it with chili, parsley, lemon juice, salt, pepper and 1 tsp. olive oil.

Heat the oven to 220F.

Marinate the chicken with 1 tsp. oil, turmeric, paprika and let it rest for 10 minutes.

Heats a pan over medium heat until it is hot then add marinated chicken and allow it to cook for a minute on both sides until golden. Transfer the chicken to the oven (and bake for 8 to 10 minutes or until it is cooked through.

In a little oil, fry the ginger and red onions until they are soft and then add in the kale and sauté it for 5-10 minute until it's done.

Cook the buckwheat in 25 to 30 minutes, dress it with the chili tomato sauce and serve with kale and chicken.

Nutrition Facts: Calories: 290, Fat: 3.8g, Carbohydrate: 24.3g, Protein: 22g

Seared Tuna in Soy Sauce and Black Pepper

Preparation Time: 15 minutes

Cooking Time: 8 minutes

Servings: 1

Ingredients:

5 ounces tuna, 1-inch thick

1 red onion, chopped

2 tbsp. soy sauce

¼ tsp. ground black pepper

½ tbsp. grated ginger

1 tsp. sesame seeds

2 tsp. extra virgin olive oil

2 cups baby spinach

1 tbsp. orange juice

Directions:

Marinate tuna with 1tbsp. soy sauce, oil and black pepper for 30 minutes. Place a skillet over high heat and when very hot, add tuna and quickly cook 1 minute per side.

Cut the tuna in slices, dress them with 1 tbsp. soy sauce mixed with grated ginger. Add green onion and sesame seeds on top.

Serve with a baby spinach salad dressed with 1 tsp olive oil, salt, pepper and orange juice.

Nutrition Facts: Cal 154 Fats 4.1 g Carbohydrate 3g Protein 15 g

Sirt Salmon Salad

Preparation time: 5 minutes

Cooking time: 30 minutes

Servings: 2

Ingredients:

1 large Medjool date, thinly chopped

1 cup chicory leaves

½ cup arugula

1 tsp. of extra virgin olive oil

1 tbsp. parsley, chopped

3 oz. celery, sliced

6 walnuts, chopped

1 tbsp. capers

2 oz. red onion-sliced

½ avocado-peeled, stoned, and sliced

Juice of ¼ lemon

6 oz. smoked salmon

Directions:

Mix chicory and arugula and put them on a large plate. Evenly distribute on top finely sliced onion, avocado, walnuts, capers, celery and parsley.

Mix oil, lemon juice with a pinch of salt and pepper and distribute the dressing on top.

Nutrition Facts: Calories: 353, Fat: 4.8g, Carbohydrate: 28.1g, Protein: 28.3g

Green Veggies Curry

Preparation Time: 15 minutes.

Cooking Time: 25 minutes

Servings: 2

Ingredients:

3 tbsp. coconut oil

¼ small red onion, chopped

1 tsp. garlic, minced

1 tsp. fresh ginger, minced

1 cup broccoli florets

1 tbsp. red curry paste or powder

2 cups spinach

½ cup coconut cream

2 tsp. low-sodium soy sauce

½ chili

1 tsp. fresh parsley, chopped finely

Directions:

In a large skillet, melt 2 tbsp. of the coconut oil over medium-high heat and sauté the onion for about 3-4 minutes. Add the garlic, chili and ginger and sauté for about 1 minute. Add the broccoli and stir to combine well.

Immediately reduce the heat to medium-low and cook for about 1-2 minutes, stirring continuously.

Stir in the curry paste and cook for about 1 minute, stirring continuously. Add in the spinach and cook or about 2 minutes, stirring frequently.

Add the coconut cream and remaining coconut oil and stir until smooth.

Stir in the soy sauce and simmer for about 5-10 minutes, stirring occasionally or until curry reaches the desired thickness.

Remove from the heat and serve hot, topped with parsley.

Nutrition Facts: Calories 324 Fat 24.5 g Carbs 8 g Protein 17.5 g

Shrimp Tomato Stew

Preparation time: 35--40 minutes

Cooking time: 20--30 minutes

Servings: 1

Ingredients:

8 oz. shrimps

1 tbsp. extra virgin olive oil

2 leeks, finely chopped

1 large carrot, finely chopped

1 celery stick, finely chopped

1 Garlic clove, finely chopped

1 Bird's eye chili, thinly sliced

2 tbsp. wine

2 cups tomatoes

2 cups stock

1 tbsp. parsley, chopped

Salt and pepper to taste

Directions:

Fry garlic, onion, celery, carrot and chili with oil over a low heat for 5 minutes. Add the leeks. Turn up the heat to medium, add the wine and let evaporate.

Add tomatoes and cook for 5 minutes, then add the stock and let simmer for 20 minutes.

Add shrimps and let cook for 4-5 minutes until they become opaque. Don't overcook.

Serve warm.

Nutrition Facts: Calories: 213 Cal Fat: 13.1 g Protein: 80.62 g Sugar: 51.67 g

Turkey Breast with Peppers

Preparation Time: 5 Minutes

Cooking time: 25 Minutes

Servings: 2

Ingredients:

4 oz. buckwheat

8 oz. turkey breast

1 tsp. ground turmeric

2 peppers, chopped

2 oz. red onion, sliced

1 oz. celery

1 tsp. chopped fresh ginger

1 lemon, juiced

2 tsp. extra virgin olive oil

1 large tomato

1 chili, finely chopped

1 oz. parsley, finely chopped

Directions:

Boil the buckwheat 25 minutes then drain. Set aside. In the meantime, marinate the turkey breast with turmeric, 1tsp oil, lemon juice, celery and ginger.

Cook the marinated chicken in the oven for 10 to 12 minutes. Remove from the oven, cover with foil, and leave to rest for 5 minutes before serving. Meanwhile, fry the red onions and the ginger in a1 tsp oil, until they become soft, then add peppers and fry on high heat for 6 minutes. They have to stay crunchy. Serve buckwheat alongside chicken and peppers.

Nutrition Facts: Calories 107 Total Fat 2.9 g Total Carbs 20.6 g Protein 2.1 g

Goat Cheese Salad with Cranberries and Walnut

Preparation time: 20 minutes

Cooking time: 30 minutes

Servings: 2

Ingredients:

2 tbsp. dried cranberries

10 walnuts, chopped

1 cup lettuce

½ cup arugula

½ cup baby spinach

1 tbsp. balsamic vinegar

1 tsp mustard

4 oz. goat cheese

2 tsp extra virgin olive oil

Salt and pepper to taste

Directions:

Mix lettuce, arugula and baby spinach. Whisk oil, mustard, salt, pepper and vinegar, put the dressing on the salad and mix well.

Transfer to a serving plate. Crumble goat cheese over.

Add cranberries and walnuts on top and serve.

Nutrition Facts: Calories: 250 Fat: 20.9g Protein: 20.3g Carbohydrate: 3.4g

Spicy Chicken Stew

Preparation time: 10 minutes

Cooking time: 30 minutes

Servings: 2

Ingredients:

2 red peppers, chopped	1 tbsp. paprika
2 large onion, sliced	1 chili, sliced
2 garlic cloves, minced	1 tomato, chopped
1 ½ cups vegetable broth	4 chicken tights
3 tsp. extra virgin olive oil	4 oz. buckwheat
½ tsp. ground nutmeg	1 tbsp. parsley

Directions:

Boil the buckwheat for 25 minutes then drain it and set it aside.

Put the oil in a pan and heat, add onion, garlic, chili and spices and cook for 5 minutes until soft. Add the chicken and let it turn golden brown on medium high heat for 5 minutes.

Add the peppers and the tomato, salt and pepper and cook another 3-5 minutes until they start soften. Add the stock, turn the heat down and let simmer for 25 minutes. Add the buckwheat and let it absorb all the spicy flavors for 2-3 minutes. Serve hot.

Nutrition Facts: Calories: 305, Fat: 9.5g, Carbohydrate: 14.2g, Protein: 3.7g

Chapter 11.   Week 2 – Phase 2 Recipes

Fluffy Blueberry Pancakes

Preparation time: 5 minutes

Cooking time: 15 minutes

Servings: 2

Ingredients:

1 egg

2 oz. self-raising flour

1 oz. buckwheat flour

1/3 cup skimmed milk

1 cup blueberries

2 tsp honey

Directions:

Mix the flours in a bowl, add the yolk and a bit of mix in a very thick batter. Keep adding the milk bit by bit to avoid lumps.

In another bowl, beat the egg white until stiff and then mix it carefully to the batter.

Put enough batter to make a 5-inch round pancake to cook 2 minutes per side until done. Repeat until all the pancakes are ready.

Put 1 tsp. honey and ½ cup blueberries on top of each serving.

Nutrition Facts: Calories: 272, Fat: 4.3g, Carbohydrate: 26.8g, Protein: 23.6g

Caprese Skewers

Preparation time: 5 minutes

Cooking time: 30 minutes

Servings: 2

Ingredients:

4 oz. cucumber, cut in 8 pieces

8 cherry tomatoes

8 small balls of mozzarella or 4 oz. mozzarella cut in 8 pieces

1 tsp. of extra virgin olive oil

8 basil leaves

2 tsp. of balsamic vinegar

salt and pepper to taste

Directions:

Use 2 medium skewers per person or 4 small ones. Alternate the ingredients in the following order: tomato, mozzarella, basil, yellow pepper, cucumber and repeat.

Mix oil, vinegar, salt and pepper and pour the dressing over the skewers.

Nutrition Facts:

Calories: 280 kcal, Fat: 8.6g, Carbohydrate: 14.4g, Protein: 17.2g

Baked Salmon with Stir Fried Vegetables

Preparation time: 20 minutes

Cooking time: 30 minutes

Servings: 2

Ingredients:

Grated zest and juice of 1 lemon

1 tsp. sesame oil

2 tsp. extra virgin olive oil

2 carrots cut into matchsticks

Bunch of kale, chopped

2 tsp. of root ginger, grated

8 oz. wild salmon fillets

Salt and pepper to taste

Directions:

Mix ginger lemon juice and zest together. Place the salmon in an oven proof dish and pour over the lemon ginger mixture. Cover with foil and leave for 30-60 minutes to marinate.

Bake the salmon at 375°F in the oven for 15 minutes. While cooking heat up a wok or frying pan then add sesame oil and olive oil. Add the vegetables, and cook, stirring constantly for a few minutes.

Once the salmon are cooked spoon some of the salmon marinade onto the vegetables and cook for a few more minutes. Serve the vegetables onto a plate and top with salmon.

Nutrition Facts: Calories 458kcal, Fat 13.2 g Carbohydrate 15.3 Protein 21.4

Kale and Mushroom Frittata

Preparation time: 15 minutes

Cooking time: 30 minutes

Servings: 4

Ingredients:

8 eggs

½ cup unsweetened almond milk

Salt and ground black pepper, to taste

1 tbsp. extra virgin olive oil

1 red onion, chopped

1 garlic clove, minced

1 cup fresh mushrooms, chopped

1½ cups fresh kale, chopped

Directions:

Preheat oven to 350ºF. In a large bowl, place the eggs, coconut milk, salt, and black pepper, and beat well. Set aside. In a large ovenproof pan, heat the oil over medium heat and sauté the onion and garlic for about 3–4 minutes. Add the kale salt, and black pepper, and cook for about 8–10 minutes.

Stir in the mushrooms and cook for about 3–4 minutes. Place the egg mixture on top evenly and cook for about 4 minutes, without stirring. Transfer the pan in the oven and bake for about 12–15 minutes or until desired doneness.

Remove from the oven and let rest for about 3–5 minutes before serving.

Nutrition Facts: Calories 151, Total Fat 10.2 g, Total Carbs 5.6 g, Protein 10.3 g

Trout with Roasted Vegetables

Preparation time: 25 minutes

Cooking time: 20 minutes

Servings: 2

Ingredients:

2 turnips, peeled and chopped

Extra virgin olive oil

Dried dill

1 lemon, juiced

2 carrots cut into sticks

2 parsnips, peeled and cut into wedges

2 tbsp. Tamari

2 trout fillets

Directions:

Put the sliced vegetables into a baking tray. Sprinkle with a dash of tamari and olive oil. Set on gas mark 7 in the oven. Take the vegetables out of the oven after 25 minutes, and stir well.

Put the fish over it. Sprinkle with the dill and lemon juice. Cover with foil, and go back to the oven.

Turn down the oven to 375°F and cook till the fish is cooked through for 20 minutes.

Nutrition Facts: Calories 154.0 Total Fat 2.2 g Carbohydrate 14.5 Protein 23.6

Banana Strawberry Smoothie

Preparation time: 5 minutes

Servings: 1

Ingredients:

1 cup strawberries

½ banana

½ cup almond milk, unsweetened

½ tsp cocoa powder

3 cubes ice (optional)

Directions:

Blend all ingredients together and serve immediately.

Nutrition Facts:

Calories: 92kcal, Fat: 1.3g, Carbohydrate: 12.8g, Protein: 3.6g

Mince Stuffed Peppers

Preparation Time: 15 minutes

Cooking Time: 60 minutes

Servings: 4

Ingredients:

4 oz. lean mince

¼ cup brown rice, cooked

2 large yellow

2 red bell peppers

1 tbsp. parmesan

2 tbsp. breadcrumbs

3 oz. mozzarella

1 egg

¼ cup walnuts, chopped

Salt and pepper, to taste

2 cups Arugula

2 tsp. extra virgin olive oil

Few drops Lemon juice

Cooking spray

Directions:

Preheat oven to 350 degrees F.

In a bowl mix mince, parmesan, brown rice, egg and mozzarella. Mix well and set aside.

Cut peppers lengthwise, remove the seeds, fill them with the mince mix and put them on a baking tray.Distribute breadcrumbs on top and lightly spray with cooking spray to have a crunchy top without adding calories to the recipe.

Cook for 50-60 minutes until peppers are soft. Let cool for a few minutes.

Serve stuffed peppers with an arugula salad dressed with olive oil, salt and a few drop of lemon.

Nutrition Facts: Calories 375.1 Fat 8.2g Carbohydrate 24.7g Protein 15.3g

Vanilla Parfait with Berries

Preparation time: 5 minutes

Cooking time: 0 minutes

Servings: 1

Ingredients:

4 oz. Greek yogurt

1 tsp honey or maple syrup

1 cup mixed berries, frozen is perfect

1 tbsp. buckwheat granola

½ tsp Vanilla extract

Directions:

Mix yoghurt, vanilla extract and honey. Alternate yogurt and berries in a jar and top with granola.

Frozen berries are perfect if the parfait is made in advance because they release their juices in the yoghurt.

As far as granola, you can use a tablespoon of the one on page 88.

Nutrition Facts:

Calories: 318, Fat: 5.4g, Carbohydrate: 22.8g, Protein: 21.9g

Arugula Salad with Turkey and Italian Dressing

Preparation time: 5 minutes

Cooking time: 30 minutes

Servings: 2

Ingredients:

8oz. turkey breast

1 cup arugula

1 cup lettuce

2 tsp. Dijon mustard

1 tbsp. cumin

1/2 cup celery, finely diced

2 tsp. oregano

1/4 cup scallions, sliced

2 tsp. extra virgin olive oil

Salt and pepper to taste

Directions:

Grill the turkey and shred it. Set aside.

Mix lettuce and arugula on a plate. Evenly distribute shredded turkey, celery and scallions.

In a small bowl mix all dressing ingredients: mustard, oil, lemon juice, oregano, salt and pepper and pour it over the salad just before serving.

Nutrition Facts: Calories: 165 kcal, Fat: 2.9g, Carbohydrate: 13.6g, Protein: 26.1g

Creamy Mushroom Soup with Chicken

Preparation Time: 10 minutes

Cooking Time: 40 minutes

Servings: 3

Ingredients:

2 cups vegetable stock

8 oz. mixed mushrooms, sliced

1 red onion, finely diced

1 carrot, finely diced

1 stick celery, finely diced

4 oz. chicken breast, cubed

1 tbsp. extra virgin olive oil

3 leaves sage

Directions:

Put 1 tbsp. oil in a skillet and cook chicken until lightly brown. Set aside.

Put the mushrooms in a hot pan with 1 tbsp. oil, celery, carrot, onion and sage and cook for 3 to 5 minutes.

Add the stock and let it simmer for another 5 minutes, then using a hand blender, blend the soup until smooth.

Add the chicken and cook for another 8 to 10 minutes until creamy.

Nutrition Facts: Calories 302.0 Fat 3.5 g Carbohydrate 16.3 Protein 15 g

Super Easy Scrambled Eggs and Cherry Tomatoes

Preparation time: 2 minutes

Cooking time: 2 minutes

Servings: 1

Ingredients:

2 Eggs

1 tbsp. Parmesan or other shredded cheese

Salt and pepper

½ cup cherry tomatoes

Directions:

Put eggs and cheese with a pinch of salt and pepper in a jar. Microwave for 30 seconds, then quickly stir with a spoon.

Put back in the microwave for 60 seconds and they are a ready to eat with cherry tomatoes.

In case you don't own a microwave, cook the scrambled eggs in a skillet for 2 minutes, stirring continuously until done.

Nutrition Facts: Calories: 278, Fat: 5.4g, Carbohydrate: 12.8g, Protein: 18.9g

Lemon Ginger Shrimp Salad

Preparation time: 15 minutes

Cooking time: 5 minutes

Servings: 2

Ingredients:

1 cup chicory leaves

½ cup arugula

½ cup baby spinach

2 tsp. of extra virgin olive oil

6 walnuts, chopped

1 avocado-peeled, stoned, and sliced

Juice of ½ lemon

8 oz. shrimps

1 pinch chili

Directions:

Mix chicory, baby spinach and arugula and put them on a large plate.

Heat a skillet on medium high temperature, put 1 tbsp. oil and cook shrimps with garlic, chili, salt and pepper until they are not transparent anymore (5 minutes)

Blend avocado with oil, lemon juice with a pinch of salt and pepper and distribute the dressing on top. Chop the walnuts, put them on the plate as last ingredient and serve.

Nutrition Facts: Calories: 353, Fat: 4.8g, Carbohydrate: 28.1g, Protein: 28.3g

Blueberry Smoothie

Preparation time: 5 minutes

Servings: 1

Ingredients:

1 cup blueberries

½ banana

½ cup orange juice

3 cubes ice (optional)

Directions:

Blend all ingredients together and serve immediately.

Nutrition Facts: Calories: 87, Fat: 1.1g, Carbohydrate: 11.8g, Protein: 1.6g

Lemon Chicken Skewers with Peppers

Preparation time: 5 minutes

Cooking time: 15 minutes

Servings: 8

Ingredients:

8 oz. chicken breast

2 cups peppers, chopped

1 cup tomatoes, chopped

3 tsp. extra virgin olive oil

1 garlic clove

½ lemon, juiced

½ tsp paprika

½ tsp turmeric

1 handful parsley, chopped

Salt and pepper

Directions:

Cut the breast in small cubes and let it marinate with oil and spices for 30 minutes.

Prepare the skewers and set aside.

Heat a pan with oil. When hot add garlic and cook 5 minutes, the remove the clove.

Add peppers, tomatoes, salt and pepper and cook on high heat for 5-10 minutes.

Heat another pan to high heat, when very hot, put the skewers in and cook 10-12 minutes until golden on every side. Serve the skewers alongside the peppers.

Nutrition Facts: Calories: 315 Fat: 20.9g Protein: 15.8g Carbohydrate: 5.4g

Overnight Oats with Strawberries and Chocolate

Preparation time: 5 minutes + 8h

Cooking time: 0 minutes

Servings: 2

Ingredients:

2 oz. rolled oats

4 oz. almond milk, unsweetened

2 tbsp. plain yoghurt

1 cup strawberries

1 tsp honey

1 square 85% chocolate

Directions:

Mix the oats and the milk in a jar and leave overnight. In the morning top the jar with yoghurt, honey, strawberries and chocolate cut in small pieces.

It can be prepared in advance and left up to 3 days in the fridge.

Nutrition Facts: Calories: 258, Fat: 3.3g, Carbohydrate: 29.8g, Protein: 13.6g

Spicy Salmon with Turmeric and Lentils

Preparation Time: 5 Minutes

Cooking time: 30 Minutes

Servings: 4

Ingredients:

Skinned salmon

1 tsp. extra virgin olive oil

1 tsp. turmeric

1/4 juice of a lemon

½ red onion, finely chopped

3 oz. lentils, canned

1 garlic clove, finely chopped

1 bird's eye chili, finely chopped

5 oz. celery cut into 2cm sticks

1 tsp. Mild curry powder

1 large tomato, cut into 8 wedges

1 cup chicken or vegetable stock

1 tbsp. parsley, chopped

Directions:

Heat the oven to 400°F. Heat a frying pan over a medium–low heat; add the olive oil, then onion, garlic, ginger, chili, and celery. Fry gently for 2–3 minutes or until softened, then add the curry powder and cook for another minute.

Add the tomatoes, then stock and lentils, and simmer gently for 10 minutes. You may want to increase or decrease the cooking time depending on how crunchy you like your celery.

Meanwhile, mix the turmeric, oil, and lemon juice and rub over the salmon. Place on a baking tray and cook for 8–10 minutes. To finish, spread parsley on top of the celery and serve with the salmon.

Nutrition Facts: Calories: 177kcal Carbohydrates: 4g Protein: 12g

Chicken and Broccoli Creamy Casserole

Preparation time: 15 minutes

Cooking time: 30 minutes

Servings: 2

Ingredients:

3 cups broccoli

8 oz. chicken breast, cubed

1/2 onion

1 cup mushrooms

½ cup broth

2 tbsp. wine

1 tbsp. flour

2 tbsp. Parmesan

Directions:

Heat the oven to 350°F. Steam the broccoli for 5 minutes, drain and cool in water and ice to set the bright green color.

Cut the chicken breast in medium sized cubes. Mix chicken and broccoli and put them in a baking tray.

Prepare the creamy sauce. Sauté the onion with olive oil on a low heat, then set to high heat, put in the mushrooms, a pinch of salt and pepper, flour and mix.

Add the wine and mix until it has evaporated. Add the broth, cook for 5 minutes, then hand blend until smooth.

Pour the sauce over the chicken and broccoli, spread 2 tbsp. of Parmesan and cook in the oven for 30-35 minutes. Turn on the broiler for the last 5 minutes.

Nutrition Facts: Calories: 353, Fat: 4.8g, Carbohydrate: 28.1g, Protein: 28.3

Sautéed Mushrooms and Poached Eggs

Preparation time: 10 minutes

Cooking time: 15 minutes

Servings: 2

Ingredients:

2 eggs

1 onion, sliced

1 tsp. extra virgin olive oil

10 oz. mushrooms, sliced

10 oz. tomatoes, chopped

1 tsp marjoram (or thyme)

Directions:

Sauté the onions in a frying pan with the oil for 5 minutes. Add mushrooms, tomatoes, herbs and season with salt and pepper to taste.

While the mushrooms are cooking, bring some water to a boil, crack one egg per time and poach it. Put the poached egg on top of mushrooms and serve.

Nutrition Facts: Calories: 270, Fat: 4.3g, Carbohydrate: 19.8g, Protein: 22.8g

Asian Beef Salad

Preparation time: 15 minutes

Cooking time: 8 minutes

Servings: 2

Ingredients:

3 tsp. extra virgin olive oil

8 oz. sirloin steaks

½ red onion, finely sliced

½ cucumber, sliced

½ cup cherry tomatoes, halved

2 cups lettuce

1 handful parsley

1 tbsp. soy sauce

½ bird's eye chili

3 tbsp. lemon juice

Directions:

Crush the garlic, mix it with finely sliced chili and parsley, 2 tsp olive oil and soy sauce. This will be the dressing.

Prepare the salad in a bowl placing lettuce on the bottom, then onion, cherry tomatoes and cucumber. Heat a skillet until very hot. Brush the steaks with remaining oil, season them with salt and pepper and cook them to your taste.

Transfer the steaks onto a cutting board for 5 minutes before slicing. Drizzle the dressing on the salad and mix well. Place steak slices on top and serve.

Nutrition Facts: Calories 262, Total Fat 12 g , Total Carbs 15.2 g Protein 25.2 g

Chocolate Mousse

Preparation time: 5 minutes

Servings: 1

Ingredients:

½ avocado

1 tsp cocoa powder

1 tsp honey

Directions:

Blend all ingredients together and serve immediately.

Nutrition Facts: Calories: 87, Fat: 1.1g, Carbohydrate: 11.8g, Protein: 1.6g

Creamy Turkey and Asparagus

Preparation time: 10 minutes

Cooking time: 30 minutes

Servings: 2

Ingredients:

8 oz. turkey breast

2 cups asparagus

2 cloves garlic

½ red onion

½ bird's eye chili

2 tsp extra virgin olive oil

½ cup full fat coconut milk

Salt and pepper

Directions:

Heat a skillet over medium high heat, put oil, onion, garlic, chili and let cook for 5 minutes.

Add turkey, cut in strips, and cook it another 5 minutes until golden on all sizes. Add the asparagus, cut in 2-inch pieces and after 2 minutes add the coconut milk.

Let it simmer for 25 minutes until the sauce is creamy.

Nutrition Facts: Calories: 353, Fat: 4.8g, Carbohydrate: 28.1g, Protein: 28.3g

Banana Vanilla Pancake

Preparation time: 10 minutes

Cooking time: 15 minutes

Servings: 2

Ingredients:

1 Egg

1 Egg White

1 Banana

2 tsp honey

1 cup Rolled Oats

¼ tsp Baking Powder

A pinch of salt

1 tsp Vanilla extract

½ cup almond milk, unsweetened

Directions:

Put half banana, eggs, oats, vanilla, baking powder, salt and almond milk in a blender and blend until smooth.

Heat a skillet and when hot but batter in to form pancakes.

Top with honey and the other half banana.

Nutrition Facts: Calories: 232, Fat: 5.3g, Carbohydrate: 22.8g, Protein: 18.6g

Shredded Chicken Bowl

Preparation Time: 10 minutes

Cooking time: 35 minutes

Servings 2

Ingredients:

8 oz. chicken breast

1tsp. onion powder

1 tsp. garlic powder

2 cups broth

2 cups baby spinach

½ Lime

2 tsp extra virgin olive oil

2 ripe avocados

1 cup cherry tomatoes

Directions:

Put the chicken breasts in a saucepan with salt, pepper, onion and garlic powder. Add the broth, bring to a boil and cook 30 to 40 minutes with a lid until the meat starts to shred.

Remove the chicken from the broth move the chicken and shred it with a fork. Put the baby spinach as base in a serving bowl.

Add the shredded chicken into the bowl, sliced avocado and cherry tomatoes.

Prepare the dressing with lime, oil, salt and pepper and drizzle it over the salad just before serving.

Nutrition Facts: Calories 420, Fat: 5.6g, Carbohydrate 12.5 g, Protein: 21.4

Indian Vegetarian Meatballs

Preparation time: 5 minutes

Cooking time: 30 minutes

Servings: 2

Ingredients:

1 cup cauliflower

1 cup brown rice

¼ cup breadcrumbs

1 egg

½ tsp. turmeric

1 tsp. smoked paprika

1 tsp. of extra virgin olive oil

1 cloves garlic crushed

1 cup tomato sauce

Broth (if needed)

Cooking spray

1 tbsp. extra virgin olive oil

1 ½ tbsp. garam masala

1 tsp ginger

1 tbsp. parsley, chopped

1 red onion-diced

6oz full fat coconut milk

Directions:

Steam cauliflower for 5 minutes then blend it with rice. Use pulse in order to get a result similar to mince. Add egg, breadcrumbs, 1 clove garlic, salt, pepper, turmeric, paprika and finely chopped parsley.

Mix well until you can form meatballs. Not: if it's too dry, add 1 tbsp. egg white and mix. If it's too runny, add 1 tbsp. breadcrumb and mix. Spray a pan with cooking spray, heat it and gently cook the meatballs for 5 minutes until golden. Be careful when you turn them so that they don't break. Put them aside

In a different pan, put oil, onion ginger garlic salt and pepper and cook on low heat until the onion is done, add tomato sauce and coconut milk and let it simmer around 15 minutes until dense. Put the meatballs in the sauce and cook another 5 minutes before serving.

Nutrition Facts: Calories: 412, Fat: 7.8g, Carbohydrate: 39.1g, Protein: 18.3g

Chapter 12.   Week 3 – Phase 2 Recipes

Blueberry and Walnut Bake

Preparation time: 5 minutes

Cooking time: 30 minutes

Servings: 4

Ingredients:

4 oz. rolled oats

12 oz. almond milk, unsweetened

1 banana, ripe and mashed

½ tsp. vanilla extract

1 oz. walnuts, chopped

1 cup blueberries

To serve: ½ cup plain yoghurt

Directions:

Heat the oven to 400°F.

Mix the oats, milk, vanilla, banana, blueberries and walnuts in a bowl. Put on a baking tray lined with parchment paper and cook around 30 minutes.

It can be eaten alone or served with ½ cup plain yoghurt.

Nutrition Facts: Calories: 308, Fat: 5.3g, Carbohydrate: 35.8g, Protein: 15.6g

Shrimp Tomato Stew: Find recipe on page 121

Buckwheat Granola

Preparation time: 15 minutes

Cooking time: 30 minutes

Servings: 10

Ingredients:

2 cups buckwheat, puffed

¾ cup pumpkin seeds

¾ cup walnuts, chopped

1 tsp. ground cinnamon

1 ripe banana, mashed

2 tbsp. honey

2 tbsp. coconut oil

Directions:

Preheat your oven to 350°F. In a bowl, place the buckwheat groats, pumpkin seeds, walnuts, cinnamon and vanilla and mix well. Add banana, honey and coconut oil to the buckwheat mixture and mix until well combined.

Transfer the mixture onto a baking tray and spread in an even layer. Bake for about 25–30 minutes, stirring once halfway through.

Remove the baking tray from oven and set aside to cool.

Nutrition Facts: Calories 252 Total Fat 14.3 g Total Carbs 27.6 g Protein 7.6 g

Turkey Bacon Fajitas

Preparation time: 5 minutes

Cooking time: 20 minutes

Servings: 2

Ingredients:

3 eggs, lightly beaten

2 wholegrain tortillas

½ cup cherry tomatoes

1 red onion

2 turkey bacon slices

2 oz. cup shredded cheddar

1 tsp extra virgin olive oil

Directions:

Sauté the onion with olive oil on medium heat for 5 minutes, add the eggs and stir continuously until they are done.

Add turkey bacon, finely sliced and cheddar cheese on top so that it starts to melt.

Quick heat the tortillas on a pan (keep them soft), divide the egg mixture between them and serve immediately.

Nutrition Facts: Calories: 353, Fat: 4.8g, Carbohydrate: 28.1g, Protein: 28.3g

Brussels Sprouts Egg Skillet

Preparation time: 5 minutes

Cooking time: 30 minutes

Servings: 2

Ingredients:

½lb Brussels sprouts, halved

1 red small onion, chopped

10 cherry tomatoes, halved

4 eggs

1 tsp. extra virgin olive oil

Directions:

In an 8 inch cast iron skillet, heat olive oil over medium heat.

Add in onion and sauté for 1-2 minutes.

Add in Brussels sprouts and tomatoes and season with salt and pepper to taste.

Cook for 3-4 minutes then crack the eggs, cover and cook until egg whites have set, and egg yolk is desired consistency.

Nutrition Facts: Calories: 194, Net carbs: 18.2g, Fat: 11.4g, Protein: 7.1g

Orange Cumin Sirloin

Preparation time: 5 minutes + 8h

Cooking time: 10 minutes

Servings: 2

Ingredients:

8 oz. sirloin

2 cloves garlic, crushed

2 tbsp. extra virgin olive oil

½ lime juice

½ orange juice

¼ cup parsley

½ tsp cumin

½ bird's eye chili

2 tbsp. soy sauce

Salt and pepper

Directions:

Prepare the marinade combining all the ingredients, reserve 2 tbsp. for later and put the rest on the sirloin in a small tray. Turn the meat several times so that the marinade covers it completely. Cover with aluminum foil and put in the fridge for 8 hours.

Drain the meat from the marinade; pat it with kitchen paper in order to dry it.

Heat the grill or a skillet until very hot and cook to your taste. Let the cooked meat sit on a plate for 5 minutes then slice it and dress it with the 2 tablespoons of marinade you kept aside.

Nutrition Facts: Calories: 353, Fat: 4.8g, Carbohydrate: 28.1g, Protein: 28.3g

Simple Arugula Salad

Preparation Time: 10 minutes.

Cooking Time: 0 minutes

Servings: 4

Ingredients:

1 white onion, peeled and chopped

1 tbsp. vinegar

1 bunch baby arugula

¼ cup walnuts, chopped

2 tbsp. fresh cilantro, chopped

2 garlic cloves, peeled and minced

2 tbsp. extra virgin olive oil

1 tbsp. lemon juice

Directions:

In a bowl, mix the water and vinegar, add the onion, set aside for 5 minutes, and drain well. In a salad bowl, mix the arugula with the walnuts and onion, and stir.

Add the garlic, salt, pepper, lemon juice, cilantro, and oil, toss well, and serve.

Nutrition Facts: Calories 200 Fat 2 g Carbs 5 g Protein 7 g

Garlic Salmon with Brussel Sprouts and Rice

Preparation time: 5 minutes

Cooking time: 30 minutes

Servings: 2

Ingredients:

8 oz. salmon fillet slices

1 clove garlic, crushed

2 tbsp. wine

1 cup Brussel sprouts

1 cup cherry tomatoes

1 tsp extra virgin olive oil

3 oz. basmati rice

3 tbsp. stock (or water), if needed

Directions:

Boil the basmati rice until tender and set aside.

Crush the garlic and coat the top of the salmon. Put a skillet on medium high heat and when hot put the salmon fillets skin down. Cook for 5 minutes than turn them. Cook them until it becomes brown and crispy (around 5-6 more minutes).

Remove the salmon from the pan and add Brussel sprouts, tomatoes, wine and salt and cook them around 10 minutes. Add stock or water if needed. When done, add the basmati rice and mix to combine the flavors. Add the parmesan and serve putting the salmon on top.

Nutrition Facts: Calories: 353, Fat: 4.8g, Carbohydrate: 28.1g, Protein: 28.3g

Banana Vanilla Pancake: Find this recipe on page 144

Indian Vegetarian Meatballs: Find great recipe on page 146

Blueberry Smoothie: Find this recipe on page 137

Sesame Glazed Chicken with Ginger and Chili Stir-Fried Greens

Preparation time: 10 minutes

Cooking time: 25 minutes

Servings: 4

Ingredients:

1 mirin	1 tsp. fresh ginger
1tbsp. miso paste	1 cup spinach
6 oz. chicken breast	2 tsp. sesame seeds
1 oz. celery	3 oz. buckwheat
2 oz. red onion	1 tsp. ground turmeric
2 zucchini	1 tsp. extra virgin olive oil
1 Thai chili	1 tsp. tamari
2 garlic cloves	

Directions:

Heat the oven to 400 F. Line a roasting pan with parchment-paper Mix in the mirin and the miso. Lengthwise cut the chicken and marinate it with the miso mix for 15 minutes.

Place the chicken in the roasting pan, sprinkle it with the sesame seeds, and roast in the oven for 15 to 20 minutes until it has been beautifully caramelized.

Wash the buckwheat in a sieve, and then place it along with the turmeric in a saucepan of boiling water. Cook 25-30min until done, and then drain. Chop celery, red onion, and zucchini to medium pieces. Chop the chili, garlic, and ginger very thinly, and set aside.

Heat the oil in a frying pan; add the celery, onion, zucchini, chili, garlic, and ginger and fry over high heat for 1 to 2 minutes, then reduce to medium heat for 3 to 4 minutes until the vegetables are cooked through, but are still crunchy.

If the vegetables begin to stick to the pan, you can need to add a cup of water. Add the tamari and spinach, and cook for 2 minutes. Serve with chicken and buckwheat.

Nutrition Facts: Calories: 417, Fat: 6.5g, Carbohydrate: 34.8g, Protein: 32.1g

Super Easy Scrambled Eggs and Cherry Tomatoes Find this recipe on page 135

Brussels Sprouts and Ricotta Salad

Preparation time: 15 minutes

Cooking time: 0 minutes

Servings: 2

Ingredients:

1 ½ cups Brussel sprouts, thinly sliced

1 green apple cut "à la julienne"

½ red onion

8 walnuts, chopped

1 tsp extra virgin olive oil

1 tbsp. lemon juice

1 tbsp. orange juice

4 oz. ricotta cheese

Directions:

Put the red onion in cup and cover it with boiling water. Let it rest 10 minutes, then drain and pat with kitchen paper. Slice Brussel sprouts as thin as you can, cut the apple à la julienne (sticks).

Mix Brussel sprouts, onion and apple and season them with oil, salt, pepper, lemon juice and orange juice and spread it on a serving plate.

Spread small spoons of ricotta cheese over the serving plate and top with chopped walnuts.

Nutrition Facts: Calories: 353, Fat: 4.8g, Carbohydrate: 28.1g, Protein: 28.3g

Sesame Tuna with Artichoke Hearts

Preparation time: 5 minutes

Cooking time: 30 minutes

Servings: 2

Ingredients:

8 oz. tuna steaks

2 tbsp. white sesame

2 tbsp. black sesame

1 tsp sesame oil

2 artichokes

2 tsp extra virgin olive oil

½ lemon, juiced

1 clove garlic

1 handful parsley

Directions:

Discard the outer leaves, and then slice artichokes very finely. Heat a pan with olive oil, put garlic and cook for a couple of minutes, then remove the clove. Add artichokes, lemon, salt pepper and cook 5-10 minutes until tender. Set aside.

Mix sesame seeds and press them on tuna until it is completely covered.

Heat a pan, add sesame oil and when it's very hot cook tuna 1-2 minutes per side.

Serve tuna alongside artichokes.

Nutrition Facts: Calories: 353, Fat: 4.8g, Carbohydrate: 28.1g, Protein: 28.3g

Fluffy Blueberry Pancakes: Find this recipe on page 125

Baked Salmon with Stir Fried Vegetables: Find this recipe on page 127

Chocolate Mousse: Find this recipe on page 142

Spicy Stew with Potatoes and Spinach

Preparation time: 10 minutes

Cooking time: 30

Servings: 2

Ingredients:

2 sweet potatoes

2 tsp. extra virgin olive oil

1 red onion, finely chopped

½ bird's eye chili

2 tbsp. paprika

1 cup tomatoes, chopped

1 cup stock

1 cup spinach

8 oz. chicken breast

Salt and pepper to taste

Directions:

Peel and cut sweet potatoes in 1-inch cubes and boil them 12 minutes. Drain and set aside.

Heat a pan on medium high heat, add onion and cook for 5 minutes.

Add chicken cubes and spices and let the meat color on all sides for 5 minutes.

Add tomatoes and stock and let cook 15 minutes on low heat.

Add sweet potatoes and spinach, let mix the flavors 5 minutes then turn the heat off.

Let rest 10 minutes then serve.

Nutrition Facts: Calories: 213 Cal Fat: 13.1 g Protein: 80.62 g Sugar: 51.67 g

Sautéed Mushrooms and Poached Eggs: Find this recipe on page 141

Roasted Butternut and Chickpeas Salad

Preparation time: 15 minutes

Cooking time: 35 minutes

Servings: 2

Ingredients:

1 cup chickpeas, drained

2 cups kale

2 tsp oil

½ lemon, juiced

2 cloves of garlic

1 green apple

½ tsp honey

Salt and pepper to taste

Directions:

Heat the oven at 400°F.

Cut the squash into medium cubes, put them in a baking tray, add drained chickpeas, garlic 1 tbsp. oil, salt and pepper and mix. Cook for 25 minutes.

Mix the kale with the dressing: salt, pepper, lemon, olive oil and honey so that while the squash is cooking it becomes softer and more pleasant to eat.

When squash and chickpeas are done, put them aside 10 minute and in the meantime chop the apple and mix it with kale.

Add squash and chickpeas on top and serve warm.

Nutrition Facts: Calories: 353, Fat: 4.8g, Carbohydrate: 28.1g, Protein: 28.3g

Eggplant Pizza Towers

Preparation time: 15 minutes

Cooking time: 40 minutes

Servings: 2

Ingredients:

1 ½ eggplants	½ cup mozzarella
1 tbsp. tomato paste	4 basil leaves
2 cups tomato sauce	1 tsp extra virgin olive oil
½ red onion	1 tbsp. Parmesan
1 clove garlic	Salt and pepper

Directions:

Cut the eggplants into thick slices, add some salt and let them rest so that they let their bitter water out. In the meantime prepare the salsa. Heat a pan with oil, when hot add onion and garlic and cook 5 minutes.

Add tomato sauce, tomato paste, salt and pepper and cook on low heat for about 15-18 minutes. Add a few leaves of basil. Pat the eggplants with kitchen paper and grill them. Heat the oven at 350°F.

Compose the towers: put a slice of eggplant, sauce, a few dices of mozzarella and again eggplant, sauce, mozzarella. Three layers per tower are best. Distribute parmesan on top.

When done, put the tray in the oven for about 10 minutes until the mozzarella is melted.

Nutrition Facts: Calories: 353, Fat: 4.8g, Carbohydrate: 28.1g, Protein: 28.3g

Vanilla Parfait with Berries: Find this recipe on page 132

Arugula Salad with Turkey and Italian Dressing: Find this recipe on page 133

Mango Mousse with Chocolate Chips

Preparation time: 5 minutes

Servings: 1

Ingredients:

1 cup mango

½ cup Greek yoghurt

¼ tsp vanilla extract

2 squares dark chocolate, chopped

Directions:

Blend mango, yoghurt and vanilla together, add chocolate chips and serve immediately.

Nutrition Facts: Calories: 87, Fat: 1.1g, Carbohydrate: 11.8g, Protein: 1.6g

Greek Frittata with Garlic Grilled Eggplant

Preparation time: 5 minutes

Cooking time: 30 minutes

Servings: 2

Ingredients:

1 ½ cups shredded zucchini	1 eggplant
3 eggs	2 tbsp. oil
3 oz. feta cheese	1 clove garlic, crushed
2 tbsp. milk	1 tsp. balsamic vinegar
2 leaves mint, finely chopped	Salt and pepper to taste

Directions:

Heat the oven to 350°F. Cut the eggplant into thin slices; mix with a pinch of salt and let rest.

Mix the shredded zucchini with a pinch of salt and let it rest in a colander until they lost some water. After 10 minutes, squeeze them out and put them in a bowl.

Add 3 eggs, crushed feta cheese, milk, salt, pepper, mint, whisk well and pour in a silicone baking tray and cook 25-30 minutes in the oven. Pat the eggplant slices dry and grill them.

Mix garlic, oil, salt, pepper and balsamic vinegar and pour the dressing on the eggplants. Serve the frittata alongside the eggplant.

Nutrition Facts: Calories: 359, Fat: 7.8g, Carbohydrate: 18.1g, Protein: 21.3g

Week 4 – Transition - Recipes

Brussels Sprouts Egg Skillet: Find this recipe on page 150

Chocolate Mousse: Find this recipe on page 142

Creamy Turkey and Asparagus: Find this recipe on page 143

Spicy Indian Dahl with Basmati Rice

Preparation time: 10 minutes

Cooking time: 15 minutes

Servings: 1

Ingredients:

- 1 tsp. of extra virgin olive oil
- 2 oz. onion, nicely chopped
- 2 garlic cloves, nicely chopped
- 1 tsp. fresh ginger
- 1 chili, nicely chopped
- 1 tsp. of mild curry powder
- tsp. of ground turmeric
- 1tsp cinnamon stick
- ½ tsp. cardamom seeds
- ½ tsp. cumin seeds
- 1 cup red lentils
- 1 medium tomato, chopped
- 1 oz. basmati rice
- 1 tsp. extra virgin olive oil

Directions:

Cook the lentils in boiling water for 20 to 25 minutes until almost done. In the meantime, cook the rice in a separate pot for 20 minutes and drain.

Put cinnamon, onion, garlic, ginger, and chili in a hot pan with olive oil. Cook until tender, for about 5 minutes then discard the cinnamon. Drain the lentils and put them in the pan.

Add tomato, turmeric, curry, cardamom and cumin and cook for a few minutes until all the flavors have mixed together.

Serve Dahl with steamed rice.

Nutrition Facts: Calories: 272, Fat: 4.3g, Carbohydrate: 26.8g, Protein: 23.6g

Vanilla Parfait with Berries: Find this recipe on page 132

Lemony Chicken Burgers

Preparation time: 10 minutes

Cooking time: 10 minutes

Servings: 2

Ingredients:

8 oz. chicken mince

¼ onion, finely chopped

1 clove garlic, crushed

1 handful of parsley, finely chopped

Juice and zest of ¼ lemon

2 leaves Lettuce

½ tomato

2 tsp extra virgin olive oil

2 whole wheat buns

Directions:

Put chicken mince, onion, garlic, parsley, salt pepper, lemon zest and juice in a bowl and mix well. Form 2 patties and let rest 5 minutes.

Heat a pan with olive oil and when very hot cook 3 minutes per part. They are also very good when grilled, if you opt for grilling, just brush the patties with a bit of oil right before cooking.

Put the patties in the buns with lettuce and tomato and enjoy.

Nutrition Facts: Calories: 353, Fat: 4.8g, Carbohydrate: 28.1g, Protein: 28.3g

Walnut Energy Bar

Preparation time: 15 minutes

Cooking time: 20 minutes

Servings: 4

Ingredients:

4 oz. rolled oats

1 oz. shredded coconut

8 walnuts, chopped

½ cup almond milk, unsweetened

3 tbsp. honey

1 pinch salt

½ tsp vanilla extract

1 tbsp. peanut butter

Directions:

Mix all the ingredients, put them on a baking tin lined with parchment paper and cook 20-25 minutes at 325°F until golden and crisp.

Nutrition Facts:

Calories: 192, Fat: 4.3g, Carbohydrate: 32.8g, Protein: 6.6g

Sesame Tuna with Artichoke Hearts: Find this recipe on page 156

Baked Sweet Potato

Preparation time: 5 minutes

Cooking time: 50 minutes

Servings: 1

Ingredients:

1 medium sweet potato   1 tsp butter

Directions:

Heat the oven to 425°C.

Clean the potato very well under running water to get rid of the dirt.

Prick it several times and put it in the oven for 50minutes. Always remember to test if it's done using a stick.

Make a cut in the upper part and put the butter over.

Nutrition Facts: Calories: 353, Fat: 4.8g, Carbohydrate: 28.1g, Protein: 28.3g

Blueberry and Walnut Bake: Find this recipe on page 147

Mango Mousse with Chocolate Chips: Find this recipe on page 160

Shredded Chicken Bowl: Find this recipe on page 145

Creamy Broccoli and Potato Soup

Preparation time: 5 minutes

Cooking time: 30 minutes

Servings: 3

Ingredients:

3 cups broccoli, chopped

2 potatoes, peeled and chopped

1 large onion, chopped

3 garlic cloves, minced

1 cup raw cashews

3 cups vegetable broth

3 tsp. extra virgin olive oil

½ tsp. ground nutmeg

Directions:

Soak cashews in a bowl with boiling water and let rest for at least 4 hours.

Drain them and blend them with 1 cup of vegetable broth until smooth. Set aside. This will make the soup super creamy.

Gently heat olive oil in a large saucepan over medium-high heat. Cook onion and garlic for 3-4 minutes until tender. Add in broccoli, potato, nutmeg and water.

Cover and bring to the boil, then reduce heat and simmer for 20 minutes, stirring from time to time. Remove from heat and stir in cashew mixture.

Blend until smooth, return to pan and cook until heated through.

Nutrition Facts: Calories: 305, Fat: 9.5g, Carbohydrate: 14.2g, Protein: 3.7g

Chickpea Fritters

Preparation time: 5 minutes

Cooking time: 30 minutes

Servings: 3

Ingredients:

1 can chickpeas, drained

2 chicken breasts, cooked and shredded

2 egg whites

½ cup fresh parsley leaves, very finely cut

1 tsp. ginger

½ tsp. black pepper salt, to taste

2 tbsp. coconut oil, for frying

Directions:

Blend the chickpeas in a food processor and combine them with the chicken, egg whites, parsley, and ginger into a smooth batter.

Heat the oil in a frying pan over medium heat. Using a large spoon, scoop the batter into fritters.

Cook each one for 2-3 minutes each side or until golden and cooked through.

Nutrition Facts: Calories: 207, Net carbs: 35.6g, Fat: 3.1g, Protein: 10.3g

Lemon Tuna Steaks with Baby Potatoes

Preparation time: 5 minutes

Cooking time: 30 minutes

Servings: 2

Ingredients:

10 oz. tuna steaks

12 oz. baby potatoes, chopped

1 garlic clove, crushed

1 tbsp. thyme

½ tbsp. oregano

1 tbsp. rosemary

1 lemon

2 tsp. extra virgin olive oil

Salt and pepper to taste

Directions:

Heat the oven to 400°F. Marinate the tuna for 20 minutes with 1 tsp oil, herbs, salt, pepper and the juice of half lemon. Chop the baby potatoes and season them with oil, salt, pepper and rosemary.

Put potatoes in a baking tray, spreading the potatoes so that they are in a single layer. Cook them for 12 minutes. Cut the remaining half lemon in slices in put them on the tuna steaks. Take the tray out of the oven and add tuna steaks. Cook for another 10 minutes and serve immediately.

Nutrition Facts: Calories: 305, Fat: 5.5g, Carbohydrate: 34.2g, Protein: 23.7g

Chocolate Mousse: Find this recipe on page 142

Lamb, Butternut Squash and Date Tagine

Preparation time: 15 minutes

Cooking time: 1 hour 15 minutes

Servings: 4

Ingredients:

2 tbsp. extra virgin olive oil

1 red onion, chopped

1-inch ginger, grated

3 garlic cloves, crushed

1 tsp. chili flakes

2 tsp. cumin seeds

1 cinnamon stick

2 tsp. ground turmeric

16 oz. lamb shoulder, cut into pieces

½ tsp. salt

2 oz. dates, pitted and sliced

2 cups tomatoes

1 cup broth

2 cups butternut squash, cubed

1 can chickpeas, drained

2 tbsp. fresh coriander

1 cup basmati rice

Directions:

Heat the oven at 325°F. Add oil into a tagine pot or an ovenproof saucepan with lid, heat on low heat and when hot gently cook the onions until they are soft.

Add the grated ginger and garlic, chili, cumin, cinnamon and turmeric. Stir well and cook 1 minute. Add a dash of water if it becomes too dry. Add the lamb and stir to coat it with spices and onions. Add dates, tomatoes and 1 cup broth.

Bring the tagine into the boil, set the lid and place on your preheated oven for about 1 hour and 15 minutes. Steam the basmati rice and put aside. After 45 minutes, add butternut squash and drained chickpeas to the tagine. Stir everything together, place the lid back on and go back to the oven for 30 minutes.

Serve with basmati rice on the side.

Nutrition Facts: Calories: 380 Cal Fat: 13.1 g Protein: 80.62 g Sugar: 51.67 g

Fluffy Blueberry Pancakes: Find this recipe on page 125

Lemon Ginger Shrimp Salad: Find this recipe on page 136

Mince Stuffed Peppers: Find this recipe on page 131

Overnight Oats with Strawberries and Chocolate: Find this recipe on page 138

Chicken and Broccoli Creamy Casserole: Find this recipe on page 140

Baked Sweet Potato: Find this recipe on page 165

Buckwheat Granola: Find this recipe on page 148 and add ½ cup plain yoghurt

Spinach Quiche

Preparation time: 10 minutes

Cooking time: 40 minutes

Servings: 4

Ingredients:

5 oz. all purposes flour	1 small pinch of baking soda
2 oz. buckwheat flour	3 cups spinach
3 oz. almond flour	3 eggs
½ cup water	1 cup ricotta cheese
2 tbsp. extra virgin olive oil	1 tbsp. Parmesan

Directions:

Mix the flours, salt and baking soda. Add the water and mix until you get a dough. If needed add some more water. Let the dough rest for 30 minutes.

Heat the oven at 350°F. Heat a pan with oil, put spinach and a bit of salt and let cook 5 minutes on low heat. Set aside.

When the dough is ready, roll the dough to 1/8 Inch and put it in a baking tin. Mix ricotta, eggs, salt, pepper and spinach and put the filling in the tin.

Remove the excess dough with a knife. Bake 35 minutes. Let cool 10 minutes and serve.

Remaining dough can be stored in the fridge or freezer in an air tight container.

Nutrition Facts: Calories: 353, Fat: 4.8g, Carbohydrate: 28.1g, Protein: 28.3g

Banana Vanilla Pancake: Find this recipe on page 144

Brussels Sprouts and Ricotta Salad: Find this recipe on page 155

Energy Cocoa Balls

Preparation time: 5 minutes +30 minutes + 4 hours

Servings: 2

Ingredients:

4 dates, pitted

1 tbsp. peanut butter

20 almonds

Cocoa powder for coating

Directions:

Blend all the ingredients then put the mix in the fridge for 30 minutes. Form the balls and coat them with cocoa powder. Put them back in the fridge for 4 hours before eating.

Nutrition Facts:

Calories: 132, Fat: 5.3g, Carbohydrate: 22.8g, Protein: 4.6g

Mexican Chicken Casserole

Preparation time: 5 minutes

Cooking time: 40 minutes

Servings: 4

Ingredients:

½ cup buckwheat

½ red onion

8 oz. chicken mince

1 tbsp. paprika

½ chili

1 clove garlic

4 oz. black beans, rinsed

2 cups spinach

1 cup shredded cheddar

Directions:

Boil buckwheat for 25 minutes then rinse and put aside.

Heat a pan with oil, when hot add onion, garlic and chili and cook for 5 minutes. Add mince and spices and cook for 10 minutes stirring repeatedly. Add spinach and cook another 3 minutes.

Take a baking dish and put buckwheat as first layer, then add chicken mince.

Spread the cheese on top and bake for 10 minutes until the cheese is melted.

Nutrition Facts: Calories: 353, Fat: 4.8g, Carbohydrate: 28.1g, Protein: 28.3g

Chapter 13.   Sirtfood Diet and Workout

Sirtfood Diet is intended as your new lifestyle, not certainly a single time diet plan. For this reason, it's very important to talk not just about what you eat, but also about exercise, which is a true medicine to prevent many kind of diseases as we age.

So let's answer a common question when it comes to working out: "It possible to combine exercising during the phases of sirtfood diet, or do we need to keep workout routines out of the way?"

The answer is actually that it depends.

Especially during Phase 1, caloric intake is drastically reduced. So reducing physical activities seems the better solution for most of the people while the body to adapts to the changes. It's essential to be kind with it and support it especially the first 3 days.

After the first 3 days, though, if you already have the habit of exercising moderately all throughout the year, you can start again with exercise. It will depend on you, how far you will be able to push yourself. Just manage your fitness regime according to your diet regime and to listen to your body. In case you are feeling low in energy or if you feel fatigued, stop working out for a few days. Dedicate that time in remaining focused on the sirtfood diet principles for a healthy life.

If you never exercised before or you did but didn't built a proper habit, it's probably better if you wait until the end of Phase 2 when caloric intake will be sensibly up and it will be able to support a proper training.

It is essential to look out for a healthy way of exercising that is actually sustainable. Something that will not deprive you of enjoying your life and will not need you to keep on exercising all throughout the week.

Importance of Exercising

Proper exercising should involve all those movements that are essential in your everyday life, allowing your body to burn out calories and make muscles work in the meantime. You can opt for various types of physical exercises such as running, walking, jogging, swimming, dancing, and so on. As you start being active, you will experience various benefits over your health, both mental and physical. In fact, coupling exercises with a sirtfood diet can help in shedding extra pounds and obviously moderate exercising.

Exercise Supports Metabolism

The main aim of sirtfood diet is to cut off the extra pounds from your body. As you stay inactive or indulge in less physical activities, it can result in obesity and weight gain. For understanding the overall effect of exercising on the reduction of weight, you will need to have a clear understanding of the relationship between energy expenditure and exercise.

The human body is capable of spending energy in three definite ways: exercising, food digestion, and maintenance of body functions such as breathing and heartbeat. As you start with the diet, the calorie intake will be reduced, and that will be lowering the rate of metabolism. This might result in delaying the loss of weight. On the other hand, exercising along with your diet plan can improve the metabolic rate that will help in burning down more calories. Thus, you will be able to lose more weight without any effect on your muscle mass.

It has been found that the combination of aerobic exercise and resistance training can improve the loss of fat and can also help in the maintenance of muscle mass. So, make sure that you opt for moderate exercising as soon as you can, if anything at the end of Phase 2.

Exercise Can Support Your Mood

Exercise can help in uplifting your mood. It can also deal with depression, stress, and anxiety. As you start with sirtfood diet, your body will enter a state of shock during the first few days as you will be restricting the calories suddenly. Moderate exercising can help in dealing with stress of this kind. Exercising can bring about certain changes in the brain that can regulate anxiety and stress. In fact, it can also help in improving the sensitivity of the brain for hormones such as norepinephrine and serotonin that helps in relieving depression.

Also, exercising can improve the production of the hormone endorphins that deals with positive feelings and also help people who suffer from anxiety. With moderate exercising, you will be able to be aware of your mental state. It does not matter how intensively you exercise. You will be able to benefit even from moderate exercise. As you cut down calories during the first phase of the diet, you are most likely to develop a disturbing mood. If you feel enough energy to do it, exercise can play a deep role in regulating your mood.

Exercise Improves of Energy Levels

Exercise comes with the great power of boosting your energy level. In case you are suffering from any sort of medical condition, it can help in improving your energy in that case as well. In sirtfood diet, energy is provided by the body by burning down body fat. When you couple it with proper exercise, you can improve the benefits of the same. Exercising can help in boosting the energy levels of all those people who suffer from CFS or chronic fatigue syndrome. It is possible to treat other serious illnesses like cancer with the help of proper exercise and diet.

Exercise Can Reduce Chronic Diseases

A chronic lack of physical activity, can lead to chronic diseases. Regular exercise can help improving sensitivity to insulin, body composition, and also cardiovascular fitness. It can also help in maintaining blood pressure along with the levels of body fat.

Lack of physical exercise, even for a short period, can result in the development of body fat and can also increase the overall risk of developing diabetes of type 2. Physical exercise is necessary with proper diet for reducing belly fat percentage.

Exercising Is Beneficial For Bones and Muscles

Exercise can play a beneficial role in maintaining and building strong bones and muscles. Physical type of activity such as weight lifting can help in building muscles when it is coupled with proper intake of protein. This is mainly because exercise helps in releasing certain hormones that can promote the capability of the muscles for absorbing amino acids. This ultimately helps in growing and reducing the breakdown. With growing age, people tend to lose their muscle mass along with their function. This can result in disabilities and injuries. It is essential to opt for physical activities daily for retaining the mass of the muscles at the time of following a diet. It can help in maintaining your strength with age.

Exercising can help in improving the density of the bones that can help a lot in preventing osteoporosis at a later stage in life. Exercises that involve high impacts such as running or gymnastics or sports such as basketball and soccer have shown to improve bone density at a higher rate in comparison to non-impact activities such as cycling and swimming.

Improves Skin Health

The quality of the skin can get affected by a high amount of oxidative stress on the body. Oxidative stress takes place when the antioxidant defenses of the body are unable to mend the damage that is caused to the cells by the free radicals. This can result in damaging the internal structures and can also lead to deterioration of the skin quality. It is true that exhaustive and intense physical activity can result in oxidative damage; daily moderate exercising on the other hand can improve the production of antioxidants naturally. This can help in protecting the skin cells. Similarly, exercising can help in stimulating the flow of blood and can also induce adaptations of the skin cells that contribute to delaying the occurrence of skin aging.

Improve Brain Memory and Health

It has been found that brain functioning can be improved with the help of regular exercise. Exercise can also help in protecting your memory and skills of thinking since it improves blood circulation to the brain. Regular exercise with a proper diet is even more important for older adults as the increased rate of inflammation and oxidative stress can also lead to changes in the structure of the brain along with its functioning.

Exercise Can Improve the Quality of Sleep

Regular exercise with a balanced diet can help in relaxing and having a good sleep because it helps releasing stress and also increases the temperature of the body which is directly related to the quality of sleep. Exercising can help in dealing with sleep disorders as well. You can be completely flexible regarding the type of exercise that you want to choose. It has been found that aerobic exercise, coupled with resistance training, can improve sleep.

Exercise Can Help In Reducing Pain

Chronic pain might turn out to be debilitating. But, with the help of exercise, you can deal with it very easily. Exercising helps in toning the muscles that remain inactive, and this, in turn, results in the reduction of pain. You will be able to improve your level of pain tolerance and also decrease the perception of pain with the help of daily exercise.

Chapter 14.   Mindset: A Fundamental Aspect

All diets work. But not all dieters manage to lose weight.

This concept can be applied to all fields of our life, for example, many people graduate with high marks, but few manage to get the job they dream of. Many people play basketball, but very few come to play in the NBA.

Why do some succeed, and others fail? What more do they have to those who fail?

And, returning to the world of diets, why is losing weight so difficult?

The answer is: The Mindset!

To be able to talk about it, you must first define what the mindset is. With this expression we want to refer, in general, to all that set of conditionings and beliefs that our mind has assimilated during life. This habitual mental attitude characterizes our ways of reacting and acting in certain circumstances. In a sense, we can define the mindset as our usual behavior in the face of situations that arise.

For example, a person convinced that he cannot speak publicly, will probably tend to avoid the occasions when it is necessary to show his/her skills in front of others. This determines a general insecurity, which if not addressed will take root more and more deeply in the mind, causing him/her to give up and surrender for fear of making mistakes.

This is precisely one of the reasons why it is essential to know ourselves in deep. Knowing what our limits are, our fears, our difficulties and being able to admit them is an essential step towards the possibility of overcoming them. Although they are often theoretical limits that we place ourselves when, in reality, our fears speak and make us believe that there are obstacles that cannot be overcome.

We said that the mindset is a mental setting that has taken root in each of us year after year. So how it is possible to change what seems to belong to us so deeply?

It is possible by practicing new behaviors, until our mind accepts them as the new mindset.

This step may not be so easy and immediate, and, above all, it may also happen that you do not immediately put the correct strategy into practice. This depends on the fact that there are rare times when it is possible to act already in the right and effective way. Different tactics correspond to each activity and situation.

This means that the transition to practice requires adjustments along the way. There is no definitive or right mindset in absolute and in all situations but for every occasion you will have to model your ad hoc strategies. The mindset is not a point of arrival but a process in progress, a continuous evolution of the personal way of approaching things.

Mindset for a successful diet

Once we have explained what the mindset is and how it influences our way of thinking, we can explain the part that interests us most: how to use it to carry out a successful diet.

Let's start by saying that food, from a psychological point of view, represents for man a fundamental need: pleasure.

Now, if food is related to pleasure, and if pleasure is a fundamental emotion (even one of the 4 fundamentals for our survival - the others are fear, anger and pain), in your opinion can we take the idea of depriving us of food? Of course the answer is no.

What typically happens in all diets is this: you follow them for some days and then stop. At best. In worst case, you follow them for some days and then explode in a binge that makes you recover all the pounds lost with interest.

In short, the more you deprive yourself of it, the more you desire it.

The solution

The solution is changing our behavior and in particular change our habit to make dieting feel so restrictive and unpleasant. Instead, we start making dieting as much pleasant as possible. Sirtfood Diet, with its massive list of allowed foods including chocolate and wine surely helps making our weight loss journey less deprived of the things we love.

But there's more to that. For example, let's talk about where we eat and how good it looks at the eye. For sure, it is more lovely to eat with a nice setting, than to do it with a plastic plate or a sandwich wrapped in paper. Eating outside, it's great to find a bench, a corner of greenery, or any other pleasant space. Better to do it by listening to some music or in the pleasant sound of silence, than with the TV on or, worse, continuing to work. The environment should help us appreciate the food; don't just pass it from the mouth to the stomach.

Another suggestion. As long as you finished following the 4-weeks Meal plan which actually includes many pleasant recipes and even some healthy chocolate snacks, consider that a happy healthy life cannot be achieved when continuously depriving ourselves.

You made an effort to change your eating habits and now are able to put together a weekly menu which helps you maintain your results. Just know that sometimes it's ok to give in to temptations.

From time to time, there should be spaces to enjoy the thing you may want to eat in that moment, even if it's not "healthy". An afternoon chocolate, a plate of pasta every now and then, a less restrictive Sunday ... Without exaggerating, of course, but ensuring that no food is permanently. This will be your secret weapon to maintain a long lasting result for life.

Appendix A - Frequently Asked Questions

Below a list of the most frequently asked questions, answered.

- **Do I Exercise During Phase 1?**

Regular exercise is one of the best things you can do for your health and doing some moderate exercise can improve your diet's weight loss and wellbeing. As a general rule, during the Sirtfood Diet's first seven days, we advise you to maintain your average level of exercise and physical activity. Nonetheless, we suggest staying in your usual comfort zone, as prolonged or overly intense exercise can simply put too much stress on the body during this time. Check the body. There's no need to force you during Phase 1 for more exercise; instead, let the Sirtfoods do the hard work.

- **I Am Slim — Can I Follow The Diet?**

For anyone who is underweight, we do not recommend Phase 1 of the Sirtfood Diet as you don't need to lose any more weight. Calculating your body mass index or BMI is a safe way to understand if you are underweight. You can easily calculate this by using one of the numerous online BMI calculators, as long as you know your height and weight. If your BMI is 18.5 or less, we do not suggest embarking on a diet phase 1. We would also advise caution if your BMI is between 18.5 and 20 because following the diet can mean that your BMI falls below 18.5. While many people strive to be super-skinny, the fact is that underweight may have a detrimental effect on many health factors, leading to a lower immune system, an increased risk of osteoporosis (weakening bones), and fertility issues. What you could do is following Phase 3 – Transition and also using the recipes in the book to create your own Meal Plan following the guidelines of Phase 3 that does not include a caloric restriction and helps you setting up a diet rich in sirtfoods.

- **I Am Obese — Is The Sirtfood Correct For Me?**

Of course! Join the thousands of people who already tried the diet and lost weight. You will reap the most considerable improvements in your well-being, thanks to sirtuin activation. Being obese increases the risk of many chronic health problems, yet these are the very illnesses which Sirtfoods will help you avoid.

- **I Reached My Target Weight, And Don't Want To Lose Any More — Do I Stop Sirtfoods Eating?**

First of all, congratulations on your success in terms of weight loss! With Sirtfoods, you've had great success, but it doesn't stop now. While we do not recommend further restriction on calories, your diet should still provide ample Sirtfoods. The great thing about Sirtfoods is they are a lifestyle. In terms of weight control, the best way to think of them is that they help get the body to the weight and shape it was meant to be. They work from here to sustain and keep you looking fantastic and feeling great.

- **I Take Medication — Is This Ok To Follow The Diet?**

The Sirtfood Diet is ideal for most people, but due to its powerful effects on fat burning and wellbeing, it can alter the processes of certain diseases and the drug acts recommended by your doctor.

If you suffer from a significant health condition, take prescription medications, or have any reasons to think about going on a diet, we recommend that you speak to your doctor about it. The chances for you are it will be a fine and indeed profound benefit, but it is necessary to check before starting.

- **I Am Pregnant - Can I Follow The Diet?**

If you are trying to conceive or are pregnant or breastfeeding, we do not suggest embarking on the Sirtfood Diet. It is a powerful diet for weight loss, which makes it inappropriate. Don't be put off eating plenty of Sirtfoods, though, as these are incredibly nutritious foods to be consumed as part of a balanced and varied pregnancy diet. Because of its alcohol content, you will want to avoid red wine and limit caffeinated items such as coffee, green tea, and cocoa not to exceed 200 milligrams of caffeine per day during pregnancy (one mug of instant coffee typically contains about 100 milligrams of caffeine). Recommendations do not exceed four cups of green tea a day and do avoid matcha altogether. Other than that, the benefits of having Sirtfoods in your diet are free to reap.

- **Are Sirtfoods Suitable For Children?**

The Sirtfood Diet is an intense diet for weight loss and not intended for kids. That doesn't mean that kids will miss out on the excellent health benefits provided by adding more Sirtfoods to their overall diet. Of course not all Sirtfoods are suitable for children, like red wine and coffee, but it's just common sense.

- **Will I Get A Headache Or Tired Feel During Phase 1?**

This diet can include symptoms such as mild headache or tiredness, but these effects are slight and short-lived. Of course, if the symptoms are severe or give you cause for concern, seek for medical advice promptly. Occasional mild symptoms will quickly resolve, and in a few days, most people have a renewed sense of energy, vigor, and well-being.

- **Should I Repeat Phases 1, 2 and 3?**

You can repeat Phase 1 again if you feel you need a weight-loss or a health boost. To ensure no long-term adverse effects of calorie restriction show up, you should wait at least a month before repeating it. Most people need to repeat it no more than at once every three months and keep getting amazing results. Instead, if you have gone off course, need some fine-tuning, or want a little more Sirtfood pressure, we suggest that you repeat as much as you Phase 2 and 3 that are, after all, about developing a lifelong way to feed. Remember, the

Sirtfood Diet's beauty is that it doesn't require you to feel like you're endlessly on a diet, but instead it's the foundation to develop positive lifelong dietary changes that create a lighter, leaner, healthier you.

- **Does The Sirtfood Diet Have Fiber Enough?**

Naturally, a lot of Sirtfoods are rich in fiber. Onions, endive, and walnuts are notable sources, with buckwheat and Medjool dates really standing out, meaning the fiber department is not short of a Sirtfood-rich diet. Even during Phase 1, when food consumption is reduced, most of us will still consume a fiber quantity that we are used to, particularly if we select from the menu options the recipes that contain buckwheat, beans, and lentils. However, for others known to be susceptible to intestinal problems such as constipation without higher fiber intakes, a suitable fiber supplement may be considered during Phase 1, especially days 1 to 3, which should be discussed with your health care professional.

- **Can I Eat What I Want Once I Eat Plenty Of Sirtfoods And Results Still Show?**

One of the main reasons why the Sirtfood Diet works so well in the long term is that it encourages good food rather than demonizing mediocre food. Exclusion diets just aren't effective long-term. It is true that processed foods high in sugars and fats decrease sirtuin activity in the body, thus reducing the benefits of Sirtfoods by high consumption. However, if you keep your attention on eating a diet rich in Sirtfoods, you will end up consuming much less garbage than the average person as a result if you are happily fulfilled and have less appetite for certain refined foods. If you sometimes indulge in these refined foods, don't worry about it — the strength of Sirtfoods, the rest of the time, will ensure that you are still reaping the benefits.

Conclusion

Congratulations, all stages of the Sirtfood Diet have now finished!

Just let's take a look of what you have achieved. You've entered the hyper-success phase 1, probably achieving a remarkable weight loss around 7 pounds and an interesting increase of muscle mass.

You also maintained your weight loss throughout the fourteen-day maintenance phase 2 and further improved your body composition. You have marked the beginning of your lifetime transformation thanks to phase 3, where you had a sample of how your new way of eating could be.

You took a stand against diseases which strikes often as we get older, enhancing your strength, productivity, and health.

By now, you are familiar with the top twenty Sirtfoods, and you've gained a sense of how powerful they are. Not only that, you probably have become quite good at including them in your diet and loving them. For the sustained weight loss and health they offer, these items must stay a prominent feature in your everyday eating regimen.

Good luck to you as you move towards the new chapter of your healthy, happy life!

Sirtfood Diet Cookbook

200 Tasty Ideas For Healthy, Quick And Easy Meals.

Enjoy The Anti Inflammatory Power Of Sirtuine Foods Combined In Delicious Recipes To Lose Weight And Feel Great In Your Body.

Kate Hamilton

Table of Contents

Introduction

It would probably surprise you, but people knew about healthy foods long before we studied them in more recent years. In ancient times, they were discovering the effects of different plants and adopt some of them in their regular diet. Of course, back then, food was natural, so they weren't dealing with the same problem as we are dealing today. Thousands of years ago, people were dying for many causes; most of them were not related to bad nutrition. They didn't have the knowledge and technology to process food. Nowadays, medicine has evolved, but bad nutrition unfortunately causes plenty of deaths.

You are probably wondering how the Sirtfood diet was discovered. The founders of this meal plan have targeted the foods with a higher concentration of sirtuin-activating nutrients. They had a hunch about what these foods can do to your body. Then based on their findings, they have analyzed the eating habits and lifestyles of different people around the world who have a diet rich in sirtuin-activating nutrients. Therefore, if the Mediterranean diet was inspired by the eating habits and lifestyle of the people living on the Mediterranean shores, the Sirtfood diet tried the same approach, but this time, the analyzed population is spread all over the world.

There are regions from all over the world called the blue zones, where people eat plenty of sirtfoods. These people have a much lower rate of Alzheimer's disease, diabetes, heart disease, osteoporosis, and even cancer. Don't be surprised if you see people in their 90s walking, working, and dancing. This probably sounds like a fairy tale, a legend, or a myth, but there are people out there who are not affected by typical "western world" lifestyle. They don't have any stress, and they are enjoying life to the fullest.

If you have the privilege of visiting the San Blas Islands of Panama, you will definitely meet the Kuna American Indians, an indigenous population with incredibly low rates of high blood pressure, diabetes, obesity, cancer, and early deaths. Do you know what their secret is? It is the consumption of cocoa, which happens to have a high concentration of sirtuin-activating nutrients. Cocoa can increase memory performance and enhance brain functionality. It works miracles when it comes to preventing diabetes and even cancer, plus it can be used for better oral hygiene, as it can protect teeth from cavities and plaque.

Let's move on to India, which used to be the jewel in the crown of the British Empire. India can be easily considered a micro-continent, as its vast territory is home to some of the most amazing veggies, fruits, plants, and spices. Speaking of spices, do you know which spice is called the "Indian solid gold"? This is turmeric, and India is responsible for more than 80 percent of the global supply. This is a frequently used condiment in Indian cuisine and a great source of curcumin, a very powerful sirtuin-activating nutrient. As it turns out, the consumption of turmeric can have anti-inflammatory and healing effects. Curcumin has even anticancer effects, so it is better to have turmeric included in your diet.

185

China can be considered the home ground for green tea, one of the drinks with the most health benefits you can find out there. People in China have been drinking green tea for more than 4,700 years, and now this beverage has become extremely popular all over the world. The consumption of green tea can be associated with a lower risk of different forms of cancer (breast, prostate, breast, or lung) or lower rates of coronary heart disease. Green tea works wonders on metabolism, and it is the perfect drink to have when you want to burn fat while keeping your existing muscle mass intact.

If you have the pleasure of traveling in the Mediterranean region, you will notice how common the extra-virgin olive oil is for their daily diet. People living in this area like to consume healthy fats, and it looks like nuts (and especially walnuts) are a good source of lipids. Their diet is designed to burn fats in the body and keep the blood sugar and insulin level to a minimum, avoiding diabetes, obesity, heart diseases, and even some forms of cancer. No wonder there are so many people from this region who are aging slowly and feeling amazing.

If you take a look over the top 20 sirtfoods, you can easily see that some of the ingredients can only come from a specific region of the world. The Sirtfood diet practically brings the whole world on your plate so that you can reap the weight loss and health benefits of the best ingredients from all over the world.

Chapter 1. Quick Recap on Sirtfood Diet

Sirtfood Diet Phases

As a newbie, it is important you understand that the Sirtfood diet does not start with a single list of ingredients in your hands. Its implementation and adaptation are more than mere selective grocery shopping. Every diet can only work effectively when we allow our body to embrace the sudden shift and change in food intake. Similarly, the Sirtfood diet also comes with two phases of adaptation. Going through these phases, leads to following the Sirtfood diet easily and successfully. After the two weight loss phases, there is a third one which is basically a maintaining phase that aims to consolidate the weight loss results in the long run.

Phase One

The first seven days of this diet plan are known as Phase One. In this phase, a dieter must focus on calorie restriction and the intake of green juices. These seven days are crucial to initiate your weight loss and usually lead to lose up to seven pounds if the diet is followed properly. If you find yourself achieving this target that means that you are on the right track.

In the first three days of the Phase One, the caloric intake is set around to 1,000 calories. While doing so, the dieter must also have green juice throughout the day, three times per day. The recipes given in the book are perfect to select from. Pick a recipe given in their respective segments and pair each with green juices.

After the first three days and for the next four days, the caloric intake is increased to 1,500 calories per day. In these four days, the green juices to drink during the day are reduced to two, paired with Sirtuin-rich food in every meal.

Phase Two

Phase Two starts right after the first week of the Sirtfood diet or Phase One. It is about going on with the diet feeling it even easier thanks to body adaptation to the new regimen. The first week enables the body to embrace the change and start working towards the weight loss goal, according to the new diet. This phase enables the body to keep losing weight slowly and steadily. Therefore, the duration of this phase is almost two weeks.

So how is this phase different from the Phase One? In this phase, there is no restriction on the caloric intake, as long as the food is rich in sirtuins and you are having 3 meals per day. As far as green juices, the intake is decreased to one per day, which will be more than enough to guarantee weight loss. You can have the juice any time in the day, even after any meal, in the morning or in the evening.

After the Diet

With the end of Phase Two comes the time which is most crucial, and that is the after-diet phase. If you haven't achieved your weight loss target by the end of phase two, then you can restart the phases all over again. Or even when you have achieved the goals but still want to lose more weight.

In any case, continue having good quality sirtfood with an everyday diet rich in sirtuin, and have green juices as a good habit. The 200 recipes in this book will help you arranging a colorful, tasty meal plan which everyone in your household will enjoy.

Chapter 2. 20 Superfood List

Main Characteristics and Benefits	Calories
Read wine is considered the first original sirtfood discovered. It contains a compound called Resveratrol, which protects the body against contracting conditions like heart attacks and cancer. When had in moderate quantities it is also responsible for weight loss in a sirtuin rich diet.	Calories: 153kcal Carbohydrate: 4.7g Protein: 0.1g Fat: 0g
Coffee is one of the most common sirtfoods known. Coffee contains a stimulant of the nervous system. Nervous system comprises of the brain and the spinal cord. Stimulation of the nervous system signals the body to break down the fat cells.	Calories: 1 kcal Carbohydrate: 0g Protein: 0.3g Fat: 0g
Kale is an important component for many effective green juices. Kale helps the body by enhancing fast and easy absorption of nutrients, making skin and hair glow, hardening nails and alkalizing the whole body.	Calories: 49 kcal Carbohydrate: 9g Protein: 4.3 g Fat: 0.9 g
Onions. They contain a large fraction of antioxidants and help reducing cell inflammation. They are also a major source of sirtuin activators that prevent and control oxidation of fatty acids in the cells.	Calories: 40 kcal Carbohydrate: 9g Protein: 1.1g Fat: 0.1g
Soy is a highly nutritious ingredient, rich in proteins, vitamins, and minerals. Regular consumption of soy in the Sirtfood diet helps in the prevention of tumors, prostate and breast cancer. Soy foods have no cholesterol and are low in saturated fatty acids	Calories: 173 kcal Carbohydrate: 9.9g Protein: 16.6g Fat: 9g
Strawberries. Fresh, juicy and sweet, they are very low in calories thanks to their high water content. Very useful in the Sirtfood diet because they are an excellent source of Vitamin C. They contain Elleagic Acid, very useful in fighting cancer and heart diseases.	Calories: 53 kcal Carbohydrate: 12.75 g Protein: 1.11g Fat: 0.50 g
Capers. They are flower buds of a small bush very common in the Mediterranean region. Rich in quercetin, they are used in	Calories: 23 kcal Carbohydrate: 4.9 g

many meat, fish and salad recipes They contain sodium, calcium, magnesium and potassium while being very low in calories. They are also rich in antioxidants	Protein: 2.4 g Fat: 0.9 g Potassium: 40 mg
Blueberries. They are a major source of minerals such as iron, phosphorous and calcium thus they are very useful to maintain healthy bones. The minerals are also important in mental health, digestion and weight loss.	Calories: 57 kcal Carbohydrate: 21.45 g Protein: 1.1 g Fat: 0.49 g
Red chicory. Rich in water and fibers, its consumption helps promoting healthy digestion, improving blood sugar control, and support weight loss by regulation of appetite. It contains a good amount of Vitamin C, Vitamin B, Vitamin K and potassium.	Calories: 20 kcal Carbohydrate 4 g Protein: 1.2 g Fat: 0 g
Medjool dates. This is an edible sweet fruit coming from the date palm tree with plenty of vitamins, minerals like potassium and phosphorus, and fiber. They help in preventing constipation and decreasing cholesterol due to soluble fiber intake.	Calories: 133 kcal Carbohydrate: 36 g. Protein: 0.8 g Fat: 0g
Parsley. It is a flowering plant rich in vitamin B, vitamin C, potassium and calcium important in reducing heart disease risk, strengthen bones and immune system. Used in many recipes, it's better to add it raw to keep its health benefits intact.	Calories: 36 kcal Carbohydrates: 6 g Protein: 3 g Fat: 0.3g
Extra virgin olive oil. It is a rich source of antioxidants and healthy fats which protect from cardiovascular diseases. Additionally, it is an important in lowering the risk of type 2 diabetes and can protect against stroke.	Calories: 119 kcal Carbohydrate: 0g Protein: 0g Fat: 13.5g.
Dark chocolate. It is a very important source of antioxidants. Flavonoids, polyphenols and tryptophan reduce the probability of heart diseases, improve brain functionality and help keeping a good mood and avoid depression.	Calories: 604 kcal Carbohydrate: 46.36 g Protein: 7.87 g Fat: 43.06 g
Matcha green tea. It is a variety of tea easy to prepare. It boosts brain and liver functionality. Catechins, have a strong antibiotic effect on the body, while potassium, Vitamin A and Vitamin C are strong antioxidant that helps in burning fat and leads to lose weight	Calories: 2.5 kcal Carbohydrate:0g Protein: 0.5g Fat:0 g

Turmeric. It is a yellow orange spice frequently used in sauces or curries for its anti-inflammatory and antioxidant properties. Rich in curcumin, it improves immune system; it protects the liver and helps digestions among many other positive benefits.	Calories: 29 kcal Carbohydrate: 6.31 g Protein: 0.91 g Fat: 0.31 g
Buckwheat. It is a seed high in fiber, essential amino acids and minerals like phosphorus, calcium, iron, copper, magnesium and potassium. It has a very low glycemic index which helps keeping blood sugar under control and it's very rich in Vitamin A and Vitamins B that help improving heart health by reducing inflammation and cholesterol levels.	Calories: 343 kcal Carbohydrate: 33 g Protein: 5.50g Fat: 1 g
Walnuts. They are a major source of fiber, healthy fats, minerals and vitamins. They are rich in antioxidants and a source of Omega-3 fats more than any other nut. They help keeping blood pressure and cholesterol low. Since they are very caloric, it's suggested to have 3-4 walnuts per day to appreciate their benefit while keeping the caloric intake under control.	Calories: 650 kcal Carbohydrate: 3.89 g Protein: 5 g Fat: 20 g
Arugula.. It is rich fibers and minerals like potassium that are very important for heart and nerve system functionality. It's also rich in calcium and can be considered one of the best vegetal sources of this mineral. Its vitamin content includes Vitamin A, B, C, and E which support liver functionality.	Calories: 2.5 kcal Carbohydrate: 0.4g. Protein: 0.3g. Fat: 0.1g.
Chili. It contains high amounts of capsaicin which has powerful anti-inflammatory effect which can impact on inflammation disorders such as arthritis. It's very high in vitamin C which is also antioxidant.	Calories: 6 kcal Carbohydrate: 1.3 g Protein: 0.3 g Fat: 0.1 g

Chapter 3. Prep Your Kitchen, Fridge and Pantry

You want this change to happen, to lose weight and finally reach your goal. So, first things first. Let's start with cleaning out the old to make room for the new.

Do a quick inventory of what is currently in your fridge and pantry: you may find several that are not compatible with the Sirtfood diet

The best thing to do would be tossing them out or give them away even if you just bought them. It's better not having around things that cannot help you reach your goal of having better health or a better-looking you.

If this is too extreme for you, or in case other people are living in your household, just put them aside at least for the very first part of the diet.

If there are others in the household, it is also important to get them on board and excited about what you are planning to accomplish so that they can either follow the same diet as you do, or at least cheer you up every day while you do your best to go towards your goal.

Essential Kitchen Tools

There are also some tools which make life easier in the kitchen, below a list of them. Our suggestion is, in case you don't have these items already, to check out garage sales and thrift shops before going to the department store: you could probably get most of them for a quarter of the price.

- Saucepans with lid - 1.5 qt. and 3 qt.
- Stockpot with lid - 6 qt.
- Nonstick skillet - 9.5" and 12"
- Cast iron skillet - at least 12"
- Set of stainless mixing bowls (s, m, l)
- Pyrex bakeware - 9x13 pan, large pie dish
- Stainless bakeware - 9x9, 9x13, 9" pie pan
- Vegetable knife (12" wedge shape blade)
- Paring knife (3" blade)
- Ladle
- Meat fork (sturdier than a regular fork)
- Spatula (variety of metal and rubber)
- Measuring spoons
- Measuring cups (1 c. and 2c.)
- Wisk
- Zester (tiny grater)

- Peppermill
- Food processor
- Microwave oven

Cooking Terms & Techniques

Poaching - Protein cooked in liquid.

Blanching - Process to trap nutrients in vegetables, kill bacteria, and lock in color. It is also a method of popping skins off of nuts.

Sweating - Cooking vegetables (usually onions and garlic) over a low heat with the lid on until translucent and limp.

Caramelizing - Vegetables, cooked at low heat in a little fat for a long time so that the natural sugars in the vegetables brown as they cook.

Sauté - A quick fry in very little fat.

Simmer - Liquid that stays just below boiling point.

Braising - A technique that uses quick hot, dry heat followed by long low heat and liquid. Pot roast is made by braising. The roast is first seared on all sides over high heat with oil only. Then the heat is reduced, and liquid is added as the roast cooks slowly to break down connective fibers (collagen) that make the meat tough.

-

200
TASTY
RECIPES

Nutritional Facts are intended per serving.

Juices and Smoothies

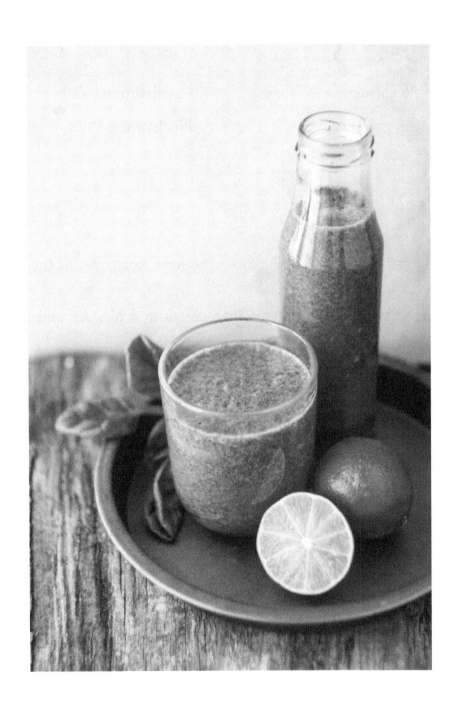

Celery Juice

Preparation Time: 10 minutes

Servings: 2

Ingredients:

8 celery stalks with leaves

2 tbsp. fresh ginger, peeled

1 lemon, peeled

½ cup filtered water

Pinch of salt

Directions:

Add all ingredients into a juicer and extract the juice according to the manufacturer's method.

In case you don't have one, add all the ingredients in a blender and pulse until well combined.

Filter the juice through a fine mesh strainer and transfer into two glasses.

Serve immediately.

Nutrition Facts: Calories 32kcal, Fat 0.5 g, Carbohydrate 6.5 g, Protein 1 g

Orange & Kale Juice

Preparation Time: 10 minutes

Servings: 2

Ingredients:

5 oranges, peeled

2 cups fresh kale

Directions:

Add all ingredients into a juicer and extract the juice according to the manufacturer's method.

In case you don't have one, add all the ingredients in a blender and pulse until well combined.

Filter the juice through a fine mesh strainer and transfer into two glasses.

Serve immediately.

Nutrition Facts: Calories 52 kcal, Fat 0.7 g, Carbohydrate 8.5 g, Protein 1.5 g

Apple, Cucumber & Celery Juice

Preparation Time: 10 minutes

Servings: 2

Ingredients:

3 apples, cored and sliced

2 cucumbers, sliced

4 celery stalks

1 1-inch piece fresh ginger, peeled

1 lemon, peeled

Directions:

Add all ingredients into a juicer and extract the juice according to the manufacturer's method.

In case you don't have one, add all the ingredients in a blender and pulse until well combined.

Filter the juice through a fine mesh strainer and transfer into two glasses.

Serve immediately.

Nutrition Facts: Calories 71kcal, Fat 0.7 g, Carbohydrate 9.2 g, Protein 1.3 g

Lemony Apple & Kale Juice

Preparation Time: 10 minutes

Servings: 2

Ingredients:

2 green apples, cored and sliced

4 cups fresh kale leaves

4 tbsp. fresh parsley leaves

1 tbsp. fresh ginger, peeled

1 lemon, peeled

½ cup filtered water

Pinch of salt

Directions:

Add all ingredients into a juicer and extract the juice according to the manufacturer's method.

In case you don't have one, add all the ingredients in a blender and pulse until well combined.

Filter the juice through a fine mesh strainer and transfer into two glasses.

Serve immediately.

Nutrition Facts: Calories 55kcal, Fat 0.3 g, Carbohydrate 6.9 g, Protein 1.2 g

Apple & Celery Juice

Preparation Time: 10 minutes

Servings: 2

Ingredients:

4 large green apples, cored and sliced

4 large celery stalks

1 lemon, peeled

Directions:

Add all ingredients into a juicer and extract the juice according to the manufacturer's method.

In case you don't have one, add all the ingredients in a blender and pulse until well combined.

Filter the juice through a fine mesh strainer and transfer into two glasses.

Serve immediately.

Nutrition Facts: Calories 62kcal, Fat 0.6 g, Carbohydrate 6.7 g, Protein 1.8 g

Apple, Orange & Broccoli Juice

Preparation Time: 10 minutes

Servings: 2

Ingredients:

2 broccoli stalks, chopped

2 large green apples, cored and sliced

3 oranges, peeled

4 tbsp. fresh parsley

Directions:

Add all ingredients into a juicer and extract the juice according to the manufacturer's method.

In case you don't have one, add all the ingredients in a blender and pulse until well combined.

Filter the juice through a fine mesh strainer and transfer into two glasses.

Serve immediately.

Nutrition Facts: Calories 82kcal, Fat 0.3 g, Carbohydrate 8.5 g, Protein 2 g

Apple, Grapefruit & Carrot Juice

Preparation Time: 10 minutes

Servings: 2

Ingredients:

3 cups fresh kale

2 large apples, cored and sliced

2 medium carrots, peeled and chopped

½ cup filtered water

2 medium grapefruit, peeled and sectioned

1 tsp fresh lemon juice

Directions:

Add all ingredients into a juicer and extract the juice according to the manufacturer's method.

In case you don't have one, add all the ingredients in a blender and pulse until well combined.

Filter the juice through a fine mesh strainer and transfer into two glasses.

Serve immediately.

Nutrition Facts: Calories 67kcal, Fat 0.2 g, Carbohydrate 8 g, Protein 0.8 g

Fruity Kale Juice

Preparation Time: 10 minutes

Servings: 2

Ingredients:

2 large green apples, cored and sliced

2 large pears, cored and sliced

3 cups fresh kale leaves

3 celery stalks

1 lemon, peeled

½ cup filtered water

Directions:

Add all ingredients into a juicer and extract the juice according to the manufacturer's method.

In case you don't have one, add all the ingredients in a blender and pulse until well combined.

Filter the juice through a fine mesh strainer and transfer into two glasses.

Serve immediately.

Nutrition Facts: Calories 65kcal, Fat 0.3 g, Carbohydrate 5.9 g, Protein 2.5 g

Green Fruit Juice

Preparation Time: 10 minutes

Servings: 2

Ingredients:

3 large kiwis, peeled and chopped

3 large green apples, cored and sliced

2 cups seedless green grapes

2 tsp fresh lime juice

½ cup filtered water

Directions:

Add all ingredients into a juicer and extract the juice according to the manufacturer's method.

In case you don't have one, add all the ingredients in a blender and pulse until well combined.

Filter the juice through a fine mesh strainer and transfer into two glasses. Serve immediately.

Nutrition Facts: Calories 105kcal, Fat 0.5 g, Carbohydrate 12.5 g, Protein 1 g

Apple & Carrot Juice

Preparation Time: 10 minutes

Servings: 2

Ingredients:

5 carrots, peeled and chopped

1 large apple, cored and chopped

1 ½-inch piece fresh ginger, peeled and chopped

½ of lemon

½ cup filtered water

Directions:

Add all ingredients into a juicer and extract the juice according to the manufacturer's method.

In case you don't have one, add all the ingredients in a blender and pulse until well combined.

Filter the juice through a fine mesh strainer and transfer into two glasses.

Serve immediately.

Nutrition Facts: Calories 125kcal, Fat 0.3 g, Carbohydrate 21.4 g Protein 1.7 g

Strawberry Juice

Preparation Time: 10 minutes

Servings: 2

Ingredients:

2½ cups fresh ripe strawberries, hulled

1 apple, cored and chopped

1 lime, peeled

Directions:

Add all ingredients into a juicer and extract the juice according to the manufacturer's method.

In case you don't have one, add all the ingredients in a blender and pulse until well combined.

Filter the juice through a fine mesh strainer and transfer into two glasses.

Serve immediately. It can be stored in the fridge in a proper container up to 3 days.

Nutrition Facts: Calories 108kcal, Fat 0.8 g, Carbohydrate 18.5 g, Protein 1.6 g

Chocolate and Date Smoothie

Preparation Time: 10 minutes

Servings: 2

Ingredients:

4 Medjool dates, pitted

2 tbsp. cacao powder

2 tbsp. flaxseed

1 tbsp. almond butter

1 tsp vanilla extract

¼ tsp ground cinnamon

1½ cups almond milk, unsweetened

4 ice cubes

Directions:

Add all ingredients in a high-power blender and pulse until smooth.

Pour into two glasses and serve immediately.

It can be stored in the fridge in a proper container up to 3 days.

Nutrition Facts: Calories 234kcal, Fat 5 g, Carbohydrate 25.5 g, Protein 6 g

Blueberry & Kale Smoothie

Preparation Time: 10 minutes

Servings: 2

Ingredients:

2 cups frozen blueberries

2 cups fresh kale leaves

2 Medjool dates, pitted

1 tbsp. chia seeds

1 ½-inch piece fresh ginger, peeled and chopped

1½ cups almond milk, unsweetened

Directions:

Add all ingredients in a high-power blender and pulse until smooth.

Pour the smoothie into two glasses and serve immediately.

It can be stored in the fridge in a proper container up to 3 days.

Nutrition Facts: Calories 230kcal, Fat 4.5 g, Carbohydrate 28.8 g, Protein 5.6 g

Strawberry & Beet Smoothie

Preparation Time: 10 minutes

Servings: 2

Ingredients:

2 cups frozen strawberries, pitted and chopped

2/3 cup frozen beets, chopped

1 ½-inch piece ginger, chopped

1 ½-inch piece fresh turmeric, chopped (or 1 tsp turmeric powder)

½ cup fresh orange juice

1 cup almond milk, unsweetened

Directions:

Add all ingredients in a high-power blender and pulse until smooth.

Pour the smoothie into two glasses and serve immediately.

It can be stored in the fridge in a proper container up to 3 days.

Nutrition Facts: Calories 130kcal, Fat 0.2g, Carbohydrate 22.5 g, Protein 2 g

Green Pineapple Smoothie

Preparation Time: 5 minutes

Servings: 1

Ingredients:

1 cup spinach

1 apple

1 cup pineapple

1tsp. of flax seeds

½ cup filtered water

Directions:

Add all ingredients in a high-power blender and pulse until smooth.

Pour the smoothie into two glasses and serve immediately.

Nutrition Facts: Calories 102kcal, Fat 0.3 g, Carbohydrate 18.5 g, Protein 1 g

Spinach Smoothie

Preparation Time: 5 minutes

Servings: 1

Ingredients:

1 cup spinach

1 pear

½ bananas

¼ zucchini

½ cup almond milk, unsweetened

Directions:

Add all ingredients in a high-power blender and pulse until smooth.

Pour the smoothie into two glasses and serve immediately.

Nutrition Facts: Calories 123kcal, Fat 0.9 g, Carbohydrate 18.5 g, Protein 2.4 g

Kale Smoothie

Preparation Time: 5 minutes

Servings: 1

Ingredients:

1 cup kale

½ mango

½ banana

1 tbsp. chia seeds

¼ cup coconut milk, unsweetened

½ cup filtered water

Directions:

Add all ingredients in a high-power blender and pulse until smooth.

Pour the smoothie into two glasses and serve immediately

Nutrition Facts: Calories 156kcal, Fat 4.5 g, Carbohydrate 20.5 g, Protein 3.2 g

Avocado Smoothie

Preparation Time: 5 minutes

Cooking Time: 0 minutes

Servings: 1

Ingredients:

½ avocado

1 banana

1 cup spinach

1 tbsp. linseed

¼ cup almond milk, unsweetened

½ cup filtered water

Directions:

Add all ingredients in a high-power blender and pulse until smooth.

Pour the smoothie into two glasses and serve immediately

Nutrition Facts: Calories 161kcal, Fat 5.5 g, Carbohydrate 29.5 g, Protein 1 g

Lettuce Smoothie

Preparation Time: 5 minutes

Servings: 1

Ingredients:

½ small head of lettuce

3 fresh plums, seeded

½ banana

1 tbsp. linseed

½ cucumber

½ cup almond milk, unsweetened

Directions:

Add all ingredients in a high-power blender and pulse until smooth.

Pour the smoothie into two glasses and serve immediately.

Nutrition Facts: Calories 138kcal, Fat 2.5 g, Carbohydrate 19.8 g, Protein 3g

Apple and Cinnamon Smoothie

Preparation Time: 5 minutes

Servings: 2

Ingredients:

2 apples, peeled, cored, sliced

4 tbsp. pecans

4 Medjool dates, pitted

½ tsp vanilla extract, unsweetened

2 cups almond milk, unsweetened

1 ½ tbsp. ground cinnamon

Directions:

Add all ingredients in a high-power blender and pulse until smooth.

Pour the smoothie into two glasses and serve immediately.

It can be stored in the fridge in a proper container up to 3 days.

Nutrition Facts: Calories 183kcal, Fat 5.5 g, Carbohydrate 12.8 g, Protein 4.5g

Strawberry, Mango and Yogurt Smoothie

Preparation Time: 5 minutes

Servings: 2

Ingredients

1 mango, destoned, peeled, diced

4 oz. strawberries

1.3 oz. yogurt

2 cups almond milk, unsweetened

Directions

Add all ingredients in a high-power blender and pulse until smooth.

Pour the smoothie into two glasses and serve immediately.

It can be stored in the fridge in a proper container up to 3 days.

Nutrition Facts: Calories 166kcal, Fat 3.7 g, Carbohydrate 27 g, Protein 3.5g

Berries Vanilla Protein Smoothie

Preparation Time: 5 minutes

Servings: 2

Ingredients:

2 oz. blackberries

2 oz. strawberries

2 oz. raspberries

2 scoops of vanilla protein powder

1 ½ cup almond milk, unsweetened

Directions:

Add all ingredients in a high-power blender and pulse until smooth.

Pour the smoothie into two glasses and serve immediately.

It can be stored in the fridge in a proper container up to 3 days.

Nutrition Facts: Calories 151kcal, Fat 2.8 g, Carbohydrate 10.9 g, Protein 20.3g

Breakfast

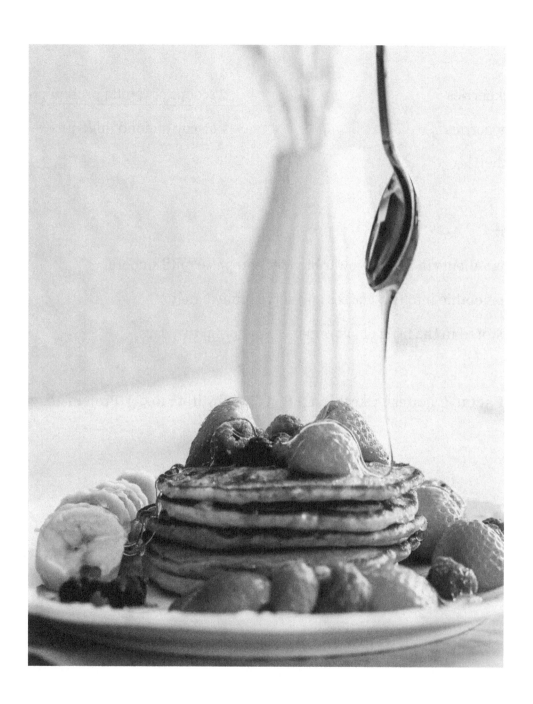

Pancakes with Apples and Blackcurrants

Preparation Time: 5 Minutes

Cooking Time: 50 Minutes

Servings: 4

Ingredients:

2 apples cut into small chunks

2 cups of quick cooking oats

1 cup flour of your choice

2 egg whites

1 ¼ cups almond milk, unsweetened

Cooking spray

1 cup blackcurrants, stalks removed

3 tbsp. water may use less

2 tbsp. raw sugar, or coconut sugar, or honey, or a few stevia drops (optional)

Directions:

Place the ingredients for the topping in a small pot simmer, stirring frequently for about 10 minutes until it cooks down and the juices are released. Take the dry ingredients and mix in a bowl.

After, add the apples and the milk a bit at a time (you may not use it all), until it is a batter. Whisk the egg whites until they are firm and gently mix them into the pancake batter.

Set aside in the refrigerator. Spray a flat pan with cooking spray, and when hot, pour some of the batter into it in a pancake shape. When the pancakes start to have golden brown edges and form air bubbles, they are ready to be flipped. Repeat for the next pancakes. Top each pancake with the berry topping.

Nutrition Facts: Calories: 370kcal, Fat: 10.83 g, Carbohydrates: 79 g, Protein: 11.71 g

Flax Waffles

Preparation Time: 5 minutes

Cooking Time: 5 minutes

Servings: 2

Ingredients

½ cup whole-wheat flour

½ tbsp. flaxseed meal

½ tsp baking powder

1 tbsp. olive oil

½ cup almond milk, unsweetened

¼ tsp vanilla extract, unsweetened

2 tbsp. raw sugar, or coconut sugar, or honey, or a few stevia drops (optional)

Directions:

Switch on a mini waffle maker and let it preheat for 5 minutes. Meanwhile, take a medium bowl, place all the ingredients in it, and then mix by using an immersion blender until smooth.

Pour the batter evenly into the waffle maker, shut with lid, and let it cook for 3 to 4 minutes until firm and golden brown.

Serve straight away. Cool the waffles, divide them between two meal prep containers, evenly add berries into the container, and then add maple syrup in mini-meal prep cups.

Cover each container with lid and store in the refrigerator for up to 5 days.

When ready to eat, enjoy them cold or reheat them in the microwave for 40 to 60 seconds or more until hot.

Nutrition Facts: Calories 220kcal, Fat 3.7 g, Carbohydrate 7 g, Protein 21.5g

Raspberries Parfait

Preparation Time: 5 minutes

Cooking Time: 0 minutes

Servings: 2

Ingredients

4 oz. raspberries

3 tbsp. chia seeds

2 ½ tbsp. shredded coconut

3 tbsp. maple syrup

8 oz. almond milk, unsweetened

½ tsp vanilla extract, unsweetened

Directions:

Take a medium bowl, place chia and coconut in it; add maple syrup and vanilla pour in the milk and whisk until well combined. Let the mixture rest for 30 minutes, then stir it and refrigerate for a minimum of 3 hours or overnight.

Assemble the parfait: divide half of the chia mixture into the bottom of serving glass, and then top evenly with three-fourth of raspberries.

Cover berries with remaining chia seed mixture and then place remaining berries on top. Serve straight away.

Use wide-mouth pint jars to layer parfait cover tightly with lids and store jars in the refrigerator for up to 7 days. When ready to eat, enjoy it cold.

Nutrition Facts: Calories 239kcal, Fat 9.5 g, Carbohydrate 9.9 g, Protein 34g

Blueberries Pancake

Preparation Time: 5 minutes

Cooking Time: 10 minutes;

Servings: 2

Ingredients

1 banana, peeled

4 tbsp. peanut butter

¼ cup whole-wheat flour

2 oz. blueberries

1 tbsp. maple syrup

A pinch of ground cinnamon

½ cup almond milk, unsweetened

Cooking spray

Directions:

Add all the ingredients in a blender and then pulse for 2 minutes until smooth. Spray a medium skillet pan with cooking spray, place it over medium heat and until it gets hot.

Pour in some batter into the pan, shape batter to form a pancake, and cook for 2 to 3 minutes per side until golden brown.

Transfer cooked pancakes to a plate and then repeat with the remaining batter. Serve straight away.

Pancakes can be stored up to 3 days in the fridge using a proper container with a lid. When ready to eat, reheat in the microwave oven for 1 to 2 minutes until hot and then serve.

Nutrition Facts: Calories 408kcal, Fat 14 g, Carbohydrate 53 g, Protein 10.2g

Cashew Biscuits

Preparation Time: 25 minutes

Cooking Time: 14 minutes

Servings: 9

Ingredients

1¼ cups whole wheat flour

⅓ cup toasted whole cashews, unsalted

½ tsp fine sea salt

1½ teaspoons baking powder

1 tbsp. coconut oil

3 tbsp. natural smooth cashew butter

½ cup soft silken tofu or unsweetened plain yogurt

Directions:

Preheat the oven to 425°F. Line a baking sheet with parchment paper. Place the flour and nuts in a food processor.

Pulse until almost all the nuts are chopped: a few larger pieces are okay and add texture to the cookies. Add salt and baking powder and pulse a couple of times.

Add oil and nut butter and pulse to combine. Add tofu or yogurt, and pulse until a crumbly (but not dry) dough forms.

Gather the dough on a piece of parchment and pat it together to shape into a 6-inch square.

Cut into nine 2-inch square biscuits. Transfer the cookies to the baking sheet. Bake for 12 to 14 minutes or until golden brown at the edges cool on a wire rack and serve.

Nutrition Facts: Calories 166kcal, Fat 3.7 g, Carbohydrate 27 g, Protein 3.5g

Raspberry Waffles

Preparation Time: 5 minutes

Cooking Time: 5 minutes

Servings: 2

Ingredients:

½ cup whole-wheat flour

1 ½ tbsp. chopped raspberry

½ tsp baking powder

1 tbsp. olive oil

½ cup almond milk, unsweetened

¼ tsp vanilla extract, unsweetened

2 tbsp. coconut sugar or a few drops of stevia (optional)

Directions:

Switch on the waffle maker and let it preheat for 5 minutes. Meanwhile, take a medium bowl, place all the ingredients in it, and then mix by using an immersion blender until smooth.

Pour the batter evenly into the waffle maker, shut with lid, and let it cook for 3 to 4 minutes until firm and golden brown.

Serve straight away. Cool the waffles, divide them between two meal prep containers, evenly add berries into the container, and then add maple syrup in mini-meal prep cups.

Cover each container with lid and store in the refrigerator for up to 5 days.

When ready to eat, enjoy them cold or reheat them in the microwave for 40 to 60 seconds or more until hot.

Nutrition Facts: Calories 229kcal, Fat 3.7 g, Carbohydrate 35.4 g, Protein 3.5g

Cherry Parfait

Preparation Time: 5 minutes

Cooking Time: 0 minutes

Servings: 2

Ingredients

3 oz. cherries, destemmed

3 tbsp. chia seeds

2 ½ tbsp. shredded coconut

3 tbsp. maple syrup

8 oz. almond milk, unsweetened

½ tsp vanilla extract, unsweetened

Directions:

Take a medium bowl, place chia and coconut in it; add maple syrup and vanilla pour in the milk and whisk until well combined.

Let the mixture rest for 30 minutes, then stir it and refrigerate for a minimum of 3 hours or overnight.

Assemble the parfait: divide half of the chia mixture into the bottom of serving glass, and then top evenly with three-fourth of cherries.

Cover berries with remaining chia seed mixture and then place remaining cherries on top. Serve straight away.

Nutrition Facts: Calories 236kcal, Fat 9.2g, Carbohydrate 34.7g, Protein 3.5g

Pancakes with Blackcurrant Compote

Preparation Time: 5 Minutes

Cooking Time: 35 Minutes

Servings: 4

Ingredients:

1 cup plain flour

½ cup porridge oats

2 apples peeled and cut into tiny pieces

1 tsp of baking powder

2 egg whites

1 cup almond milk, unsweetened

Cooking spray

Pinch of salt

4 oz. blackcurrants, stalks removed

3 tbsp. of water

2 tbsp. of raw sugar, or coconut sugar, or honey of a few drops of stevia

Directions:

Make the compote first. Place the blackcurrants, water, and sugar in a small pan. Bring it to a simmer and let it cook for 10 to 15 minutes. Place oats, baking powder, flour, and salt in a large bowl and stir well. Add in the apple then the milk a little at a time as you whisk until you have a smooth batter.

Whisk the egg whites into stiff peaks and fold into the pancake batter. Transfer the ready batter to a jug. Spray a pan with cooking spray, place it on medium high heat and add in approximately a quarter of the batter. Let it cook on both sides until it turns golden brown.

Remove when ready then repeat to make four pancakes. Drizzle the blackcurrant compote over the pancakes and serve.

Nutrition Facts: Calories 201kcal, Fat 7 g, Carbohydrate 40g, Protein 5.8g

Strawberry Buckwheat Pancakes

Preparation Time: 5 Minutes

Cooking Time: 45 Minutes

Servings: 4

Ingredients:

3½ oz. strawberries, chopped

3½ oz. buckwheat flour

1 egg

8fl oz. milk

1 tsp olive oil

1 tsp olive oil for frying

1 orange, juiced

Directions:

Pour the milk into a bowl and mix in the egg and a tsp of olive oil. Sift in the flour to the liquid mixture until smooth and creamy.

Allow it to rest for 15 minutes. Heat a little oil in a pan and pour in a quarter of the mixture or to the size you prefer.

Sprinkle in a quarter of the strawberries into the batter. Cook for around 2 minutes on each side.

Serve hot with a drizzle of orange juice.

Try this recipe with other berries such as blueberries and blackberries.

Nutrition Facts: Calories 180kcal, Fat 7.5 g, Carbohydrate 22.5 g, Protein 7.4g

Buckwheat Porridge

Preparation Time: 10 minutes

Cooking Time: 15 minutes

Servings: 2

Ingredients:

1 cup buckwheat, rinsed

1 cup almond milk, unsweetened

1 cup water

½ tsp ground cinnamon

½ tsp vanilla extract

¼ cup fresh blueberries

1 tbsp. raw honey (optional)

Directions:

In a pan, add all the ingredients (except honey and blueberries) over medium-high heat and bring to a boil.

Now, reduce the heat to low and simmer, covered for about 10 minutes. Stir in the honey and remove from the heat.

Set aside, covered, for about 5 minutes. With a fork, fluff the mixture, and transfer into serving bowls.

Top with blueberries and serve.

Nutrition Facts: Calories 358 kcal; Fat 4.7 g; Carbohydrate 3.7 g; Protein 12 g

Cherry and Vanilla Protein Shake

Preparation Time: 5 minutes

Cooking Time: 0 minutes

Servings: 1

Ingredients:

2 oz. cherries, destemmed

1 scoop vanilla protein powder

1 cup almond milk, unsweetened

Directions:

Place all the ingredients in the order into a food processor or blender, and then pulse for 1 to 2 minutes until smooth.

Serve immediately.

Nutrition Facts: Calories 193kcal, Fat 5.2 g, Carbohydrate 38 g, Protein 5.2g

Peanut Butter Cup Protein Shake

Preparation Time: 5 minutes

Cooking Time: 0 minutes

Servings: 2

Ingredients:

1 banana, peeled

1 scoop of chocolate protein powder

1 tbsp. nutritional yeast

2 tbsp. peanut butter

½ cup almond milk, unsweetened

½ tsp turmeric powder

Directions:

Place all the ingredients in the order into a food processor or blender, and then pulse for 1 to 2 minutes until smooth.

Distribute smoothie between two glasses and then serve.

Divide smoothie between two jars or bottles, cover with a lid, and then store the containers in the refrigerator for up to 3 days.

Nutrition Facts: Calories 233cal, Fat 11 g, Carbohydrate 17 g, Protein 14g

Kale Scramble

Preparation Time: 10 minutes

Cooking Time: 6 minutes

Servings: 2

Ingredients:

4 eggs

1/8 tsp ground turmeric

Salt and ground black pepper, to taste

1 tbsp. water

2 teaspoons olive oil

1 cup fresh kale, chopped

Directions:

In a bowl, add the eggs, turmeric, salt, black pepper, and water and with a whisk, beat until foamy. In a skillet, heat the oil over medium heat.

Add the egg mixture and stir to combine.

Reduce the heat to medium-low and cook for about 1–2 minutes, stirring frequently.

Stir in the kale and cook for about 3–4 minutes, stirring frequently.

Remove from the heat and serve immediately.

Nutrition Facts: Calories 183kcal, Fat 13.4 g, Carbohydrate 4.3 g, Protein 12.1 g

Tomato Frittata

Preparation Time: 10 minutes

Cooking Time: 20 minutes

Servings: 2

Ingredients:

¼ cup cheddar cheese, grated

¼ cup kalamata olives halved

8 cherry tomatoes, halved

4 large eggs

1 tbsp. fresh parsley, chopped

1 tbsp. fresh basil, chopped

1 tbsp. olive oil

1 tbsp. tomato paste

Directions:

Whisk eggs together in a large mixing bowl.

Toss in the parsley, basil, olives, tomatoes and cheese, stirring thoroughly. In a small skillet, heat the olive oil over high heat.

Pour in the frittata mixture and cook until firm (around 10 minutes).

Remove the skillet from the hob and place it under the grill for 5 minutes until golden brown.

Divide into portions and serve immediately.

Nutrition Facts: Calories 269 kcal; Fat: 23.76 g, Carbohydrate: 5.49 g, Protein: 9.23 g

Green Omelet

Preparation Time: 5 Minutes

Cooking Time: 35 Minutes

Servings: 1

Ingredients:

1 tsp of olive oil

1 shallot peeled and finely chopped

2 large eggs

Salt and freshly ground black pepper

A handful of parsley, finely chopped

A handful of rocket

Directions:

Heat the oil in a large frying pan, over medium low heat. Add the shallot and gently fry for about 5 minutes. Increase the heat and cook for two more minutes.

In a cup or bowl, whisk the eggs; distribute the shallot in the pan then add in the eggs. Evenly distribute the eggs by tipping over the pan on all sides.

Cook for about a minute before lifting the sides and allowing the runny eggs to move to the base of the pan.

Sprinkle rocket leaves and parsley on top and season with pepper and salt to taste.

When the base is just starting to brown, tip it onto a plate and serve right away.

Nutrition Facts: Calories 221 kcal, Fat 28 g, Carbohydrate 10.6 g, Protein 9.5 g

Main Dishes

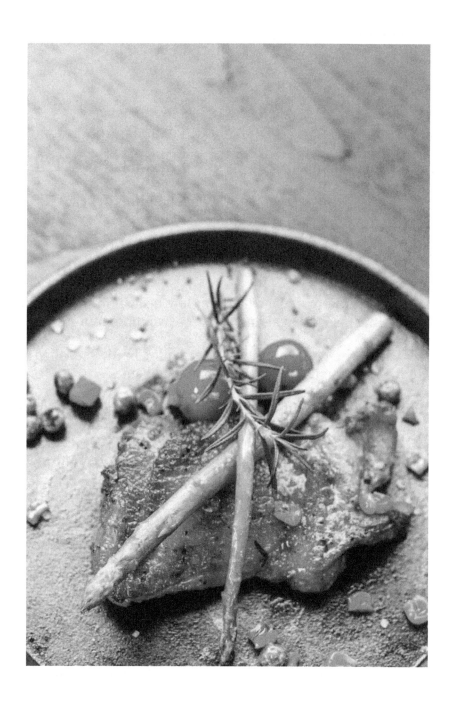

Tofu with Cauliflower

Preparation Time: 5 Minutes

Cooking Time: 45 Minutes

Servings: 2

Ingredients:

¼ cup red pepper, seeded

1 Thai chili, cut in two halves, seeded

2 cloves of garlic

1 tsp of olive oil

1 pinch of cumin

1 pinch of coriander

Juice of a half lemon

8oz tofu

8oz cauliflower, roughly chopped

1 ½oz red onions, finely chopped

1 tsp finely chopped ginger

2 teaspoons turmeric

1oz dried tomatoes, finely chopped

1oz parsley, chopped

Directions:

Preheat oven to 400 °F. Slice the peppers and put them in an ovenproof dish with chili and garlic.

Pour some olive oil over it, add the dried herbs and put it in the oven until the peppers are soft about 20 minutes).

Let it cool down, put the peppers together with the lemon juice in a blender and work it into a soft mass.

Cut the tofu in half and divide the halves into triangles.

Place the tofu in a small casserole dish, cover with the paprika mixture and place in the oven for about 20 minutes.

Chop the cauliflower until the pieces are smaller than a grain of rice. Then, in a small saucepan, heat the garlic, onions, chili and ginger with olive oil until they become transparent. Add turmeric and cauliflower mix well and heat again.

Remove from heat and add parsley and tomatoes mix well. Serve with the tofu in the sauce.

Nutrition Facts: Calories 298kcal, Fat 5 g, Carbohydrate 55 g, Protein 27.5g

Lemongrass and Ginger Mackerel

Preparation Time: 10 minutes

Cooking Time: 25 minutes

Servings: 4

Ingredients:

4 mackerel fillets, skinless and boneless

2 tbsp. olive oil

1 tbsp. ginger, grated

2 lemongrass sticks, chopped

2 red chilies, chopped

Juice of 1 lime

A handful parsley, chopped

Directions:

In a roasting pan, combine the mackerel with the oil, ginger and the other ingredients, toss and bake at 390° F for 25 minutes. Divide between plates and serve.

Nutrition Facts: Calories 251kcal, Fat 3.7 g, Carbohydrate 14 g, Protein 30g

Serrano Ham & Rocket Arugula

Preparation Time: 5 Minutes

Cooking Time: 60 Minutes

Servings: 2

Ingredients:

6oz Serrano ham

4oz rocket arugula leaves

2 tbsp. olive oil

1 tbsp. orange juice

Directions:

Pour the oil and juice into a bowl and toss the rocket arugula in the mixture. Serve the rocket onto plates and top it off with the ham.

Nutrition Facts: Calories 220kcal, Fat 7 g, Carbohydrate 7 g, Protein 33.5g

Buckwheat with Mushrooms and Green Onions

Preparation Time: 10 minutes

Cooking Time: 40 minutes

Servings: 2

Ingredients:

1 cup buckwheat groats

2 cups vegetable or chicken broth

3 green onions, thinly sliced

1 cup mushrooms, sliced

Salt and pepper to taste

2 tsp oil

Directions:

Combine all ingredients in a pot and cook on low heat for about 35-40min until the broth is completely absorbed.

Divide in two plates and serve immediately.

Nutrition Facts: Calories 340kcal, Fat 10 g, Carbohydrate 51 g, Protein 11g

Sweet and Sour Pan with Cashew Nuts:

Preparation Time: 30 minutes

Cooking Time: 0 minutes

Servings: 2

Ingredients:

2 tbsp. Coconut oil

2 pieces Red onion

2 pieces yellow bell pepper

12oz White cabbage

6oz Pak choi

1 ½oz Mung bean sprouts

4 Pineapple slices

1 ½oz Cashew nuts

¼ cup Apple cider vinegar

4 tbsp. Coconut blossom sugar

1½ tbsp. Tomato paste

1 tsp Coconut-Aminos

2 tsp Arrowroot powder

¼ cup Water

Directions:

Roughly cut the vegetables. Mix the arrow root with five tbsp. of cold water into a paste.

Then put all the other ingredients for the sauce in a saucepan and add the arrowroot paste for binding.

Melt the coconut oil in a pan and fry the onion. Add the bell pepper, cabbage, pak choi and bean sprouts and stir-fry until the vegetables become a little softer.

Add the pineapple and cashew nuts and stir a few more times. Pour a little sauce over the wok dish and serve.

Nutrition Facts: Calories: 573 kcal Fat: 27.81 g Carbohydrates: 77.91 g Protein: 15.25 g

Casserole with Spinach and Eggplant

Preparation Time: 1 hour

Cooking Time: 40 minutes

Servings: 2

Ingredients:

1 medium Eggplant

2 medium Onion

3 tbsp. Olive oil

3 cups Spinach, fresh

4 pieces Tomatoes

2 Eggs

¼ cup Almond milk, unsweetened

2 tsp Lemon juice

4 tbsp. Parmesan

Directions:

Preheat the oven to 400 ° F.   Cut the eggplants, onions and tomatoes into slices and sprinkle salt on the eggplant slices. Brush the eggplants and onions with olive oil and fry them in a grill pan.

Cook spinach in a large saucepan over moderate heat and drain in a sieve. Put the vegetables in layers in a greased baking dish: first the eggplant, then the spinach and then the onion and the tomato.

Repeat this again. Whisk eggs with almond milk, lemon juice, salt and pepper and pour over the vegetables.

Sprinkle parmesan over the dish and bake in the oven for about 30 to 40 minutes.

Nutrition Facts: Calories: 446 kcal Fat: 31.82 g Carbohydrates: 30.5 g Protein: 13.95 g

Vegetarian Curry

Preparation Time: 15 minutes

Cooking Time: 1 hour

Servings: 2

Ingredients:

4 medium Carrots

2 medium Sweet potatoes

1 large Onion

3 cloves Garlic

4 tbsp. Curry powder

½ tsp caraway, ground

½ tsp Chili powder

Sea salt to taste

1 pinch Cinnamon

½ cup Vegetable broth

1 can Tomato cubes

8oz Sweet peas

2 tbsp. Tapioca flour

Directions:

Roughly chop carrots, sweet potatoes onions potatoes and garlic and put them all in a pot.

Mix tapioca flour with curry powder, cumin, chili powder, salt and cinnamon and sprinkle this mixture on the vegetables.

Add tomato cubes. Pour the vegetable broth over it.

Close the pot with a lid, bring to a boil and let it simmer for 60 minutes on a low heat. Stir in snap peas after 30min. Cauliflower rice is a great addition to this dish.

Nutrition Facts: Calories: 397 kcal Fat: 6.07 g Carbohydrates: 81.55 g Protein: 9.35 g

Fried Cauliflower Rice:

Preparation Time: 55 minutes

Cooking Time: 10 minutes

Servings: 2

Ingredients:

1 medium Cauliflower	1 tsp Chili flakes
2 tbsp. Coconut oil	½ Carrot
1 medium Red onion	½ Red bell pepper
4 cloves Garlic	½ Lemon, juiced
¼ cup Vegetable broth	2 tbsp. Pumpkin seeds
2-inch fresh ginger	2 tbsp. fresh coriander

Directions:

Cut the cauliflower into small rice grains using a food processor.

Finely chop the onion, garlic and ginger, cut the carrot into thin strips, dice the bell pepper and finely chop the herbs. Melt 1 tbsp. of coconut oil in a pan and add half of the onion and garlic to the pan and fry briefly until translucent.

Add cauliflower rice and season with salt. Pour in the broth and stir everything until it evaporates, and the cauliflower rice is tender.

Take the rice out of the pan and set it aside. Melt the rest of the coconut oil in the pan and add the remaining onions, garlic, ginger, carrots and peppers.

Fry for a few minutes until the vegetables are tender. Season them with a little salt.

Add the cauliflower rice again, heat the whole dish and add the lemon juice.

Garnish with pumpkin seeds and coriander before serving.

Nutrition Facts: Calories: 230 kcal Fat: 17.81 g Carbohydrates: 17.25 g, Protein: 5.13 g

Buckwheat with Onions

Preparation Time: 10 minutes

Cooking Time: 40 minutes

Servings: 4

Ingredients:

3 cups of buckwheat, rinsed

4 medium red onions, chopped

1 big white onion, chopped

5 oz. extra-virgin olive oil

3 cups of water

Salt and pepper, to taste

Direction:

Soak the buckwheat in the warm water for around 10 minutes. Then add in the buckwheat to your pot. Add in the water, salt and pepper to your pot and stir well.

Close the lid and cook for about 30-35 minutes until the buckwheat is ready. In the meantime, in a skillet, heat the extra-virgin olive oil and fry the chopped onions for 15 minutes until clear and caramelized.

Add some salt and pepper and mix well. Portion the buckwheat into four bowls or mugs. Then dollop each bowl with the onions. Remember that this dish should be served warm.

Nutrition Facts: Calories: 132; Fat: 32g; Carbohydrates: 64g; Protein: 22g

Tuna, Egg & Caper Salad

Preparation Time: 5 Minutes

Cooking Time: 20 Minutes

Servings: 2

Ingredients:

3½ oz. red chicory

5oz tinned tuna, drained

3 ½ oz. cucumbers

1oz rocket arugula

6 black olives, pitted

2 hard-boiled eggs, quartered

2 tomatoes, chopped

2 tbsp. fresh parsley, chopped

1 red onion, chopped

1 stalk of celery

1 tbsp. capers

2 tbsp. extra virgin olive oil

1 tbsp. white vinegar

1 clove garlic, crushed

Directions:

Place the tuna, cucumber, olives, tomatoes, onion, chicory, celery, and parsley and rocket arugula into a bowl.

Combine olive oil, vinegar, garlic and a pinch of salt in a vinaigrette dressing.

Pour in the vinaigrette and toss the salad in the dressing. Serve onto plates and scatter the eggs and capers on top.

Nutrition Facts: Calories: 309 kcal, Fat: 12.23 g, Carbohydrates: 25.76 g, Protein: 26.72 g

Dahl with Kale, Red Onions and Buckwheat

Preparation Time: 5 Minutes

Cooking Time: 20 Minutes

Servings: 2

Ingredients:

1 tsp. of extra virgin olive oil

1 tsp. of mustard seeds

1 ½ oz. red onions, finely chopped

1 clove of garlic, very finely chopped

1 tsp very finely chopped ginger

1 Thai chili, very finely chopped

1 tsp. curry powder

2 tsp. turmeric

10 fl. oz. vegetable broth

1 ½ oz. red lentils

1 ⅝ oz. kale, chopped

1.70 fl. oz. coconut milk

1 ⅝ oz. buckwheat

Directions:

Heat oil in a pan at medium temperature and add mustard seeds. When they crack, add onion, garlic, ginger and chili. Heat until everything is soft.

Add the curry powder and turmeric, mix well. Add the vegetable stock, bring to the boil.

Add the lentils and cook them for 25 to 30 minutes until they are ready. Then add the kale and coconut milk and simmer for 5 minutes.

The dahl is ready. While the lentils are cooking, prepare the buckwheat. Serve buckwheat with the dahl.

Nutrition Facts: Calories: 273 kcal Fat: 2.41 g Carbohydrates: 24.83 g Protein: 7.67 g

Miso Caramelized Tofu

Preparation Time: 55 minutes

Cooking Time: 15 minutes

Servings: 2

Ingredients:

1 tbsp. mirin

¾ oz. miso paste

5 ¼ oz. firm tofu

1 ½ oz. celery, trimmed

1 ¼ oz. red onion

4 ¼ oz. zucchini

1 bird's eye chili

1 garlic clove, finely chopped

1 tsp. fresh ginger, finely chopped

1 ⅝ oz. kale, chopped

2 tsp. sesame seeds

1 ¼ oz. buckwheat

1 tsp. ground turmeric

2 tsp. extra virgin olive oil

1 tsp. tamari (or soy sauce)

Directions

Pre-heat your over to 400°F. Cover a tray with parchment paper. Combine the mirin and miso together. Dice the tofu and let it marinate it in the mirin-miso mixture. Chop the vegetables (except for the kale) at a diagonal angle to produce long slices.

Using a steamer, cook for the kale for 5 minutes and set aside. Disperse the tofu across the lined tray and garnish with sesame seeds. Roast for 20 minutes, or until caramelized. Rinse the buckwheat using running water and a sieve.

Add to a pan of boiling water alongside turmeric and cook the buckwheat according to the packet instructions.

Heat the oil in a skillet over high heat. Toss in the vegetables, herbs and spices then fry for 2-3 minutes. Reduce to a medium heat and fry for a further 5 minutes or until cooked but still crunchy.

Nutrition Facts: Calories: 101 kcal Fat: 4.7 g Carbohydrates: 12.38 g Protein: 4.22 g

Sirtfood Cauliflower Couscous & Turkey Steak

Preparation Time: 45 minutes

Cooking Time: 10 minutes

Servings: 2

Ingredients:

- 5 ¼ oz. cauliflower, roughly chopped
- 1 garlic clove, finely chopped
- 1 ½ oz. red onion, finely chopped
- 1 bird's eye chili, finely chopped
- 1 tsp. fresh ginger, finely chopped
- 2 tbsp. extra virgin olive oil
- 2 tsp. ground turmeric
- 1 oz. sun dried tomatoes, finely chopped
- ⅜ oz. parsley
- 5 ¼ oz. turkey steaks
- 1 tsp. dried sage
- ½ lemon, juiced
- 1 tbsp. capers

Directions:

Put the cauliflower using in the food processor and blend it in 1-2 pulses until it has a breadcrumb-like consistency.

In a skillet, fry garlic, chili, ginger and red onion in 1 tsp. olive oil for 2-3 minutes.

Throw in the turmeric and cauliflower then cook for another 1-2 minutes. Remove from heat and add tomatoes and parsley.

Marinate the turkey steak with sage, capers, lemon juice and olive oil for 10 minutes..

In a skillet, over medium heat, fry the turkey steak, turning occasionally.

Serve with the couscous.

Nutrition Facts: Calories: 462 kcal Fat: 39.86 g Carbohydrates: 9.94 g Protein: 16.81 g

Mushroom & Tofu Scramble

Preparation Time: 30 minutes

Cooking Time: 15 minutes

Servings: 1

Ingredients:

3 ½ oz. tofu, extra firm

1 tsp. ground turmeric

1 tsp. mild curry powder

¾ oz. kale, roughly chopped

1 tsp. extra virgin olive oil

¾ oz. red onion, thinly sliced

1 ⅝ oz. mushrooms, thinly sliced

A few parsley leaves, finely chopped

Directions:

Place 2 sheets of kitchen towel under and on-top of the tofu, then rest a considerable weight such as saucepan onto the tofu, to ensure it drains off the liquid.

Combine the curry powder, turmeric and 1-2 tsp. of water to form a paste. Using a steamer, cook kale for 3-4 minutes.

In a skillet, warm oil over a medium heat. Add the chili, mushrooms and onion, cooking for several minutes or until brown and tender.

Break the tofu in to small pieces and toss in the skillet. Coat with the spice paste and stir, ensuring everything becomes evenly coated.

Cook for up to 5 minutes, or until the tofu has browned then add the kale and fry for 2 more minutes. Garnish with parsley before serving.

Nutrition Facts: Calories: 333 kcal Fat: 22.89 g Carbohydrates: 18.8 g Protein: 20.9 g

Prawn & Chili Pak Choi

Preparation Time: 30 minutes

Cooking Time: 15 minutes

Servings: 1

Ingredients:

2 ¼ oz. brown rice

1 pak choi

2 fl. oz. chicken stock

1 tbsp. extra virgin olive oil

1 garlic clove, finely chopped

1 ⅝ oz. red onion, finely chopped

½ bird's eye chili, finely chopped

1 tsp. freshly grated ginger

4 ¼ oz. raw king prawns

1 tbsp. soy sauce

1 tsp. five-spice

1 tbsp. freshly chopped flat-leaf parsley

Directions:

Bring a medium sized saucepan of water to the boil and cook the brown rice for 25-30 minutes, or until softened.

Tear the pak choi into pieces. Warm the chicken stock in a skillet over medium heat and toss in the pak choi, cooking until the pak choi has slightly wilted.

In another skillet, warm olive oil over high heat. Toss in the ginger, chili, red onions and garlic frying for 2-3 minutes.

Put in the prawns, five-spice and soy sauce and cook for 6-8 minutes, or until the cooked.

Drain the brown rice and add to the skillet, stirring and cooking for 2-3 minutes. Add the pak choi, garnish with parsley and serve.

Nutrition Facts: Calories 403 kcal Fat: 15.28 g Carbohydrates: 50.87 g Protein: 16.15 g

Smoky Bean And Tempeh Patties

Preparation Time: 20 minutes

Cooking Time: 30 minutes

Servings: 4

Ingredients:

1 cup cooked cannellini beans	1 tsp smoked paprika
8 oz. tempeh	2 tbsp. organic ketchup
'¼ cup cooked bulgur	2 tbsp. maple syrup
2 cloves garlic, pressed	2 tbsp. neutral-flavored oil
¼ tsp onion powder	3 tbsp. tamari.
1 tsp liquid smoke	¼ cup chickpea flour
4 tsp Worcestershire sauce	Nonstick cooking spray

Directions:

Mash the beans in a large bowl: it's okay if a few small pieces of beans are left. Crumble the tempeh into small pieces on top. Add the bulgur and garlic.

In a medium bowl, whisk together the remaining ingredients, except the flour and cooking spray. Stir into the crumbled tempeh preparation. Add the flour and mix until well combined. Chill for 1 hour before shaping into patties.

Preheat the oven to 350°F. Line a baking tray with parchment paper. Scoop out 1/3 cup per patty, shaping into an approximately 3-inch circle and flattening slightly on the tray. You should get eight 3.5-inch patties in all. Lightly coat the top of the patties with cooking spray.

Bake for 15 minutes, carefully flip, and lightly coat the top of the patties with cooking spray and bake for another 15 minutes until lightly browned and firm.

Leftovers can be stored in an airtight container in the refrigerator for up to 4 days.

The patties can also be frozen, tightly wrapped in foil, for up to 3 months. If you don't eat all the patties at once, reheat the leftovers on low heat in a skillet lightly greased with olive oil or cooking spray for about 5 minutes on each side until heated through.

Nutrition Facts: Calories: 200kcal, Fat: 9g, Carbohydrate: 18g, Protein: 14g

Tomato & Goat's Cheese Pizza

Preparation Time: 5 Minutes + 2 hours

Cooking Time: 50 Minutes

Servings: 2

Ingredients:

8oz buckwheat flour

2 tsp. dried yeast

Pinch of salt

5fl oz. slightly water

1 tsp. olive oil

3oz feta cheese, crumbled

3oz passata or tomato paste

1 tomato, sliced

1 medium red onion, finely chopped

1oz rocket leaves, chopped

Directions:

In a bowl, combine all the ingredients for the pizza dough then allow it to stand for at least two hours until it has doubled in size.

Roll the dough out to a size to suit you. Spoon the passata onto the base and add the rest of the toppings. Bake in the oven at 400F for 15-20 minutes or until browned at the edges and crispy and serve.

Nutrition Facts: Calories: 417kcal Fat: 16g Carbohydrate: 50g Protein: 16g

Cashew Raita

Preparation Time: 10 minutes + 1 day

Cooking Time: 45 minutes

Servings: 12

Ingredients:

For the cashew base:

1 cup raw cashew pieces

¼ cup water, plus more to soak cashews, divided

¼ cup coconut cream

2 tbsp. fresh lemon juice

1 English cucumber, chopped

For the raita:

1 recipe cashew base

3 tbsp. fresh mint leaves

3 tbsp. fresh parsley

3 tbsp. fresh cilantro

2 cloves garlic, crushed

1 tsp organic lemon zest and juice

Direction:

To make the cashew base: Place the cashews in a medium bowl and cover with water.

Cover with plastic wrap, or a lid, and let stand at room temperature overnight (or about 8 hours) to soften. Drain the cashews and rinse. Put in a high-speed food processor with a cup of water, coconut cream, lemon juice, and salt.

To keep it soft, occasionally scrape the sides with a rubber spatula. This may take up to 10 minutes, depending on the power of the device. Put the cashew paste to container covered with a lid and let it sit for 24 hours at room temperature.

You will obtain a yogurt-like consistency.Chop the cucumber finely and let it rest a few minutes with a pinch of salt ultil it releases part of its water. Drain it, add the remaining ingredients and mix.

Adjust seasonings if necessary. Refrigerate for at least 2 hours or overnight to allow the flavors to melt. Leftovers can be stored in the fridge up to 4 days.

Nutrition Facts: Calories: 129.1. Fat 8.2 g Carbohydrate 13.1 g Protein 3.7 g

Green Beans With Crispy Chickpeas

Preparation Time: 30 minutes

Cooking Time: 10 minutes

Servings: 4

Ingredients:

1 can chickpeas, rinsed

1 tsp. whole coriander

1 lb. green beans, trimmed

2 tbsp. olive oil, divided

Kosher salt and freshly ground black pepper

1 tsp. cumin seeds

Grilled lemons, for serving

Directions

Heat grill to medium. Gather chickpeas, coriander, cumin, and 1 tbsp. oil in a medium cast-iron skillet. Put skillet on grill and cook chickpeas, mixing occasionally, until golden brown and coriander begins to pop, 5 to 6 minutes. Season with salt and pepper.

Transfer to a bowl. Add green beans and remaining tbsp. olive oil to the skillet. Add salt and pepper. Cook, turning once, until charred and barely tender, 3 to 4 minutes.

Toss green beans with chickpea mixture and serve with grilled lemons alongside.

Nutrition Facts: Calories: 460 Fat: 15g Carbs: 57g Protein: 16g

Sloppy Joe Scramble Stuffed Spuds

Preparation Time: 25 minutes

Cooking Time: 50 minutes

Servings: 6 potato halves

Ingredients:

1 tbsp. high heat neutral-flavored oil

1 pound extra-firm tofu, drained, pressed, and crumbled

¼ tsp fine sea salt

¼ tsp ground black pepper

¾ cup onion, finely chopped

¼ cup bell pepper (any color), finely chopped

3 cloves garlic, finely chopped

1 tbsp. ground cumin

2 tsp chili powder, or to taste

1 can (15 oz.) tomato sauce

2 tbsp. organic ketchup

1 tbsp. tamari

1 tbsp. Worcestershire sauce

1 tbsp. yellow mustard

1 4-inch dill pickle, minced

¾ cup water

3 baked potatoes, cooled

1 tbsp. olive oil

Directions:

Heat 1 tbsp. of oil in a large skillet over medium-high heat. If the skillet is not well-seasoned, add the remaining tbsp. of oil.

Add the tofu, salt, and pepper. Cook for 8 to 10 minutes, occasionally stirring until the tofu is firm and golden. Stir in the onion, bell pepper, garlic, cumin, and chili powder.

Reduce the heat to medium and cook for 3 minutes, occasionally stirring, until fragrant.

Add the tomato sauce, ketchup, tamari, Worcestershire sauce, mustard, and dill pickle. Bring to a boil, and then reduce the heat to simmer. Swish the water in the tomato sauce can to clean the sides.

Simmer for 30 minutes, occasionally stirring, adding the water from the tomato sauce can.

As needed for the desired consistency. Preheat the oven to broil. Cut the baked potatoes in half lengthwise.

Scoop the insides from the potatoes, leaving about 1 inch of the skin intact.

Brush both the insides and the outsides of the potato skins with the olive oil and place them on a baking sheet.

Broil for 3 to 4 minutes until lightly browned. Remove from the oven and divide the filling evenly in the potatoes, using about ¼ cup in each.

Nutrition Facts: Calories: 306 Fat: 21g Carbohydrate: 6g Protein: 23g

Baked Salmon Salad With Creamy Mint Dressing

Preparation Time: 20 minutes

Cooking Time: 25 minutes

Servings: 1

Ingredients:

1 salmon fillet

1 cup mixed salad leaves

1 cup lettuce leaves

Two radishes, thinly sliced

½ cucumber, sliced

2 spring onions, trimmed and chopped

½ oz. parsley, roughly sliced

For the dressing:

1 tsp low-carb mayonnaise

1 tbsp. natural yogurt

1 tbsp. rice vinegar

2 stalks mint, finely chopped

Directions:

Put the salmon fillet onto a baking tray and bake for 16--18 minutes until cooked

In a bowl, blend together the mayonnaise, yogurt, rice vinegar, mint leaves and salt and set aside 5 minutes to the flavors to mix well.

Arrange the salad leaves and lettuce onto a serving plate and top with all the radishes, cucumber, lettuce, celery, spring onions and parsley.

Drizzle the dressing.

Nutrition Facts: Calories: 433 Fat: 9g Carbohydrate: 32g Protein: 18g

Fragrant Asian Hot Pot

Preparation Time: 15 minutes

Cooking Time: 25 minutes

Servings: 2

Ingredients:

1 tsp tomato purée

1 star anise, crushed

½ oz. parsley, finely chopped

½ oz. coriander, finely chopped

Juice of 1/2 lime

2 cups chicken stock

½ carrot, cut into matchsticks

½ cup cauliflower cut into small florets

2oz beansprouts

4oz raw tiger prawns

2oz rice noodles, cooked as per packet directions

2oz cooked water chestnuts, drained

20g sushi ginger, sliced

1 tbsp. high miso paste

Directions:

Set the tomato purée, star anise, parsley stalks, coriander stalks, lime juice and chicken stock in a large pan and bring to a simmer for about 10 minutes.

Add the beansprouts, cauliflower, carrot, prawns, tofu, noodles and water chestnuts and simmer gently until the prawns are cooked.

Remove from the heat and stir at the skillet along with miso paste. Serve sprinkled with the parsley and coriander leaves.

Nutrition Facts: Calories: 397 Fat: 15g Carbohydrate: 33g Protein: 19g

Tofu Scramble With Mushrooms

Preparation Time: 15 minutes

Cooking Time: 10 minutes

Servings: 2

Ingredients:

3 tbsp. olive oil

½ yellow onion, diced

3 cloves garlic, finely chopped

1 tsp. soy sauce

12oz firm tofu, cubed

½ red bell pepper, diced

¾ cup mushrooms, cut

3 green onions, diced

2 tomatoes, cleaved

½ tsp. ground ginger

½ tsp. bean stew powder

¼ tsp. cayenne pepper

Salt and pepper to taste

Directions:

Gently sauté onion and garlic in the olive oil for 3 to 5 minutes, until they are soft. Add the remaining ingredients, except salt and pepper.

Sautee for another 6 to 8 minutes, until veggies are done and tofu absorbed the liquid. Add salt and pepper, to taste.

Nutrition Facts: Calories: 330 Fat: 9g Carbohydrate: 36g Protein: 18g

Prawn Arrabbiata

Preparation Time: 40 minutes

Cooking Time: 60 minutes

Servings: 1

Ingredients:

5oz raw prawns

2oz Buckwheat pasta

1 tbsp. extra virgin olive oil

½ Red onion, finely chopped

1 Garlic clove, finely chopped

1oz Celery, thinly sliced

1 Bird's eye chili, thinly sliced

1 tsp Dried mixed herbs

1 tsp extra virgin olive oil

2 tbsp. White wine

½ tin chopped tomatoes

1 tbsp. Chopped parsley

Directions:

Fry the garlic, onion, celery and herbs in oil on low heat for 1--2 minutes. Turn up the heat to medium, add the wine and cook until evaporated Add the tomatoes and leave the sauce simmer for 20--30 minutes, until it will reduce and get a rich texture.

While the sauce is cooking bring some water to the boil and cook the pasta as per the package directions. When cooked, drain it and put it aside.

Put prawns into the sauce and cook for a further 3--4 minutes, till they've turned opaque and pink, then add the parsley and the cooked pasta into the sauce, mix and serve.

Nutrition Facts: Calories: 335 Fat: 12g Carbohydrate: 38g Protein: 19g

Turmeric Baked Salmon

Preparation Time: 15 minutes

Cooking Time: 30 minutes

Servings: 1

Ingredients:

6 oz. Salmon fillet, skinned

1 tsp. extra virgin olive oil

1 tsp. Ground turmeric

¼ lemon, juiced

For the sauce:

1 tsp. extra virgin olive oil

1 oz. Red onion, finely chopped

1 oz. Tinned green peas

1 Garlic clove, finely chopped

1-inch fresh ginger, finely chopped

1 Bird's eye chili, thinly sliced

4 oz. Celery cut into small cubes

1 tsp Mild curry powder

1 Tomato, chopped

½ cup vegetable stock

1 tbsp. parsley, chopped

Directions:

Heat the oven to 400°F. Start cooking the sauce. Heat a skillet over a moderate --low heat, then add the olive oil then the garlic, onion, ginger, chili, celery.

Stir lightly for two --3 minutes until softened but not colored, then add the curry powder and cook for a further minute. Put in tomato, green peas and stock and simmer for 10/15 minutes depending on how thick you enjoy your sauce. Meanwhile, combine turmeric, oil and lemon juice and rub the salmon. Put on a baking tray and cook for 10 minutes in the oven. Serve the salmon with the celery sauce.

Nutrition Facts: Calories: 360 Fat: 8g Carbs: 10g Protein: 40g

Baked Potatoes With Spicy Chickpea Stew

Preparation Time: 10 minutes

Cooking Time: 60 minutes

Servings: 4

Ingredients:

4 baking potatoes, pricked around	2 tbsp. turmeric
2 tbsp. olive oil	Splash of water
2 red onions, finely chopped	2 tins chopped tomatoes
4 tsp. garlic, crushed or grated	2 tbsp. cocoa powder, unsweetened
1-inch ginger, grated	2 tins chickpeas – do not drain
1/2 tsp chili flakes	2 yellow peppers, chopped
2 tbsp. cumin seeds	2 tbsp.

Directions:

Preheat the oven to 400F; and start preparing all ingredients. When the oven is ready, put in baking potatoes and cook for 50min-1 hour until they are done.

While potatoes are cooking, put olive oil and sliced red onion into a large wide saucepan and cook lightly, using the lid, for 5 minutes until the onions are tender but not brown.

Remove the lid and add ginger, garlic, cumin and cook for a further minute on a very low heat. Then add the turmeric and a tiny dab of water and cook for a few more minutes until it becomes thicker and the consistency is ok.

Then add tomatoes, cocoa powder, peppers, chickpeas with their water and salt. Bring to the boil, and then simmer on a very low heat for 45-50 minutes until it's thick. Finally stir in the 2 tbsp. of parsley, and some pepper and salt if you desire, and also serve the stew with the potatoes.

Nutrition Facts: Calories: 520 Fat: 8g Carbohydrate: 91g Protein: 32g

Kale And Red Onion Dhal With Buckwheat

Preparation Time: 5 minutes

Cooking Time: 35 minutes

Servings: 4

Ingredients:

1 tbsp. olive oil

1 small red onion, sliced

3 garlic cloves, crushed or grated

2-inch ginger, grated

1 bird's eye chili deseeded, chopped

2 tsp. turmeric

2 tsp. garam masala

6oz snow peas

2 cups coconut milk, unsweetened

1 cup water

1 cup carrot, thinly sliced

6oz buckwheat

Directions:

Place the olive oil into a large, deep skillet and then add the chopped onion. Cook on a very low heat, with the lid for 5 minutes until softened.

Add the ginger, garlic and chili and cook 1 minute. Add turmeric and garam masala along with a dash of water and then cook for 1 minute.

Insert the snow peas, coconut milk and 1 cup water. Mix everything together and cook for 20 minutes on low heat with the lid. Stir occasionally and add a bit more water if the dhal begins to stick.

After 20 minutes add the carrot, stir thoroughly and cook for a further 5 minutes.

While the dhal is cooking, steam the buckwheat in salted boiling water for 15 minutes, drain it and serve it with the dhal.

Nutrition Facts: Calories: 340 Fat: 4g Carbohydrate: 30g Protein: 4g

Kale, Edamame And Tofu Curry

Preparation Time: 30 minutes

Cooking Time: 45 minutes

Servings: 4

Ingredients:

1 tbsp. oil

1 big onion, chopped

4 cloves garlic, peeled and grated

1 3-inch fresh ginger, peeled and grated

1 red chili, deseeded and thinly sliced

1/2 tsp. ground turmeric

1/4 tsp. cayenne pepper

1 tsp. paprika

1/2 tsp. ground cumin

1 tsp. salt

8 oz. dried red lentils

2 oz. soya edamame beans

8 oz. firm tofu, cubed

2 tomatoes, roughly chopped

Juice of 1 lime

½ cup parsley, stalks removed

Directions:

Put the oil in a pan on medium heat. When the oil is hot, add the onion and cook 5 minutes. Add ginger, garlic and chili and cook for further 2 minutes.

Add turmeric, cayenne, paprika, cumin and salt. Stir and add red lentils, soya edamame beans and tomatoes.

Pour in 4 cups boiling water and then bring to a simmer for about 10 minutes, then lower the heat and cook for a further 40 minutes until the curry becomes thicker and all flavors are blended together.

Add lime juice and parsley, stir and serve.

Nutrition Facts: Calories: 325 Fat: 6g Carbs: 77g Protein: 28g

Lemon Chicken With Spinach, Red Onion, And Salsa

Preparation Time: 30 minutes

Cooking Time: 35 minutes

Servings: 1

Ingredients:

4oz chicken breast, skinless, boneless

1 large tomato

1 chili, finely chopped

1oz capers

Juice of 1/2 lemon

2 tbsp. extra-virgin olive oil

2 cups spinach

20g red onion, chopped

2 tsp chopped garlic

3oz buckwheat

Directions:

Heat the oven to 400°F. To make the salsa, chop the tomato very finely and put it with its liquid in a bowl. The liquid is very important because it's very tasty.

Mix with chili, capers, onion, 1tbsp oil and some drops of lemon juice. Marinate the chicken breast with garlic, lemon juice and ½tbsp oil for 10 minutes.

Heat an ovenproof skillet until warm, add the chicken and cook for a minute on every side, until light gold, then move to the oven (put on a baking tray if your pan is not ovenproof) for 5 minutes until cooked.

Remove from the oven, and cover with foil. Leave to rest for 5 minutes before serving. Meanwhile, sauté the spinach for 5 minutes with ½tbsp oil and 1tbsp garlic. Serve alongside chicken with salsa and spinach.

Nutrition Facts: Calories: 342 Fat: 8g Carbs: 18g Protein: 33g

Smoked Salmon Omelet

Preparation Time: 10 minutes

Cooking Time: 15 minutes

Servings: 1

Ingredients:

2 eggs

4oz Smoked salmon, chopped

1/2 tsp. Capers

½ cup Rocket, chopped

1 tsp Parsley, chopped

1 tsp extra virgin olive oil

Directions:

Crack the eggs into a bowl and whisk well. Add the salmon, capers, rocket and parsley. Heat the olive oil in a skillet.

Add the egg mixture and, with a spatula, move the mix round the pan until it's even.

Reduce the heat and allow the omelet cook. Twist the spatula around the edges to lift them, add salmon and rocket and fold the omelet in 2.

Nutrition Facts: Calories: 303 Fat: 22g Carbohydrate: 12g Protein: 23g

Broccoli And Pasta

Preparation Time: 20 minutes

Cooking Time: 10 minutes

Servings: 2

Ingredients:

5 oz. spaghetti

5 oz. broccoli

1 garlic clove, finely chopped

3 tbsp. extra virgin olive oil

2 Shallots sliced

¼ tsp. crushed chilies

12 sage shredded leaves

Grated parmesan (optional)

Directions:

Put broccoli in boiling water for 5 minute, then add spaghetti and cook until both pasta and broccoli are done (around 8 to 10 minutes).

In the meantime, heat the oil in a frying pan and add shallots and garlic.

Cook for 5 minutes until it becomes golden.

Mix chilies and sage to the pan and gently cook for more 1 minute. Drain pasta and broccoli; mix with the shallot mixture in the pan, add some Parmesan, if desired and serve.

Nutrition Facts: Calories: 350 Fat: 8g Carbs: 38g Protein: 6g

Artichokes and Kale with Walnuts

Preparation Time: 10 minutes

Cooking Time: 30 minutes

Servings: 2

Ingredients:

1 cup of artichoke hearts

1 tbsp. parsley, chopped

½ cup of walnuts

1 cup of kale, torn

1 cup of Cheddar cheese, crumbled

½ tbsp. balsamic vinegar

1 tbsp. olive oil

Salt and black pepper, to taste

Directions:

Preheat the oven to 250°-270°Fahrenheit and roast the walnuts in the oven for 10 minutes until lightly browned and crispy and then set aside.

Add artichoke hearts, kale, oil, salt and pepper to a pot and cook for 20-25 minutes until done.

Add cheese and balsamic vinegar and stir well. Divide the vegetables in two plates and garnish with roasted walnuts and parsley.

Nutrition Facts: Calories: 152 kcal; Fat: 32g; Carbohydrates: 59g; Protein: 23g

Pecan Crusted Chicken Breast

Preparation Time: 20 minutes

Cooking Time: 35 minutes

Servings: 4

Ingredients:

½ cup whole wheat bread, dried

1/3 cup pecans

2 tbsp. Parmesan

Salt and ground pepper

1 egg white

4 chicken breasts slices, boneless and skinless (6 to 8 oz. each)

1 tbsp. grapeseed oil

Lemon cuts, for serving

1 cup mixed greens

1tbsp olive oil

Directions:

Preheat oven to 425°F. In a food processor, blitz bread, pecans and Parmesan; season with salt and pepper until you get thin breadcrumbs.

Move to a bowl. In another bowl, beat egg white until foamy. Season chicken with salt and pepper. Coat each chicken breast slice with egg white first, then put it in the breadcrumb bowl and mix until completely covered.

In a large nonstick ovenproof skillet heat grapeseed oil over medium heat. When hot, put in chicken breasts cook until gently seared, 1 to 3 minutes.

Turn chicken over and put the skillet in the oven. Cook until chicken is done (around 8 to 12 minutes). Serve chicken with lemon cuts and a plate of mixed greens with olive oil lemon and salt.

Nutrition Facts: Calories: 250 Fat: 8g Carbohydrates: 27g Protein: 17g

Tuna And Tomatoes

Preparation Time: 5 minutes

Cooking Time: 20 minutes

Servings: 4

Ingredients:

1 yellow onion, chopped

1 tbsp. olive oil

1 lb. tuna fillets, skinless and cubed

1 cup tomatoes, chopped

1 red pepper, chopped

1 tsp sweet paprika

1 tbsp. coriander, chopped

Directions:

Heat up a pan with the oil over medium heat, add the onions and the pepper and cook for 5 minutes, they have to be crispy and crunchy: don't overcook.

Add tuna, tomato and paprika and quickly cook 1 minute on high heat.

Add coriander and serve immediately..

Nutrition Facts: Calories 215 kcal, Fat 4g, Carbs 14g, Protein 7g

Tuna And Kale

Preparation Time: 5 minutes

Cooking Time: 20 minutes

Servings: 4

Ingredients:

1lb tuna fillets, skinless and cubed

A pinch of salt and black pepper

2 tbsp. olive oil

1 cup kale

½ cup cherry tomatoes, cubed

1 yellow onion, chopped

Directions:

Steam kale for 6 minutes, drizzle 1tbsp olive it and a pinch of salt and mix well.

Heat up a pan with the remaining oil over medium heat; add the onion and sauté for 5 minutes.

Add tuna and cherry tomatoes and cook for 5 minutes.

Serve the tuna with the kale on the side.

Nutrition Facts: Calories 251 kcal, Fat 4g, Carbohydrate 14g, Protein 7g

Salmon & Kale Omelet

Preparation Time: 10 minutes

Cooking Time: 7 minutes

Servings: 4

Ingredients:

6 eggs

2 tbsp. almond milk, unsweetened

Salt and ground black pepper, to taste

2 tbsp. olive oil

4 oz. smoked salmon, cut into bite-sized chunks

2 cup fresh kale, tough ribs removed and chopped finely

4 scallions, chopped finely

Directions:

In a bowl, put eggs, almond milk, salt, and black pepper, and whisk well. Set aside.

In a non-stick skillet, heat the oil over medium heat.

Place a scoop of egg mixture, distribute it evenly by rotating the skillet and cook for about 1 minute.

Place salmon kale and scallions on top of egg mixture evenly. Reduce heat to low and cook for about 4–5 minutes, or until omelet is done completely.

Carefully, transfer the omelet onto a serving plate and serve.

Nutrition Facts: Calories 210 kcal Fat 14.9 g Carbohydrates 5.2 g Protein 14.8 g

Moroccan Spiced Eggs

Preparation Time: 1 hour

Cooking Time: 50 minutes

Servings: 2

Ingredients:

1 tsp. olive oil

1 shallot, finely chopped

1 red bell pepper, finely chopped

1 garlic clove, finely chopped

1 zucchini, finely chopped

1 tbsp. tomato paste

½ tsp. mild curry

¼ tsp. ground cinnamon

¼ tsp. ground cumin

½ tsp. salt

1 can tomatoes

1 can chickpeas, drained

1/3oz parsley

4 medium eggs at room temperature

Directions:

Heat the oil in a pan; include the shallot and red bell pepper and fry on low heat for 5 minutes. Add garlic and zucchini and cook for 2 minutes. Add tomato paste, spices and salt and stir well.

Add tomatoes and chickpeas and bring to a medium heat. Put a lid on and simmer for 30 minutes until thicker. Remove from heat and add chopped parsley. Preheat the grill to 350F.

Put the tomato sauce up into a cooking tray and crack the eggs in the middle. Put the tray under the grill for 10 minutes and serve.

Nutrition Facts: Calories: 316 kcal Fat: 5.22 g Carbohydrates: 13.14 g Protein: 6.97 g

Chickpea, Quinoa And Turmeric Curry Recipe

Preparation Time: 10 minutes

Cooking Time: 1 hour

Servings: 4

Ingredients:

1lb potatoes

3 garlic cloves, squashed

3 tsp ground turmeric

1 tsp ground coriander

1 tsp mild curry

1 tsp ground ginger

2 cups coconut milk, unsweetened

1 tbsp. tomato purée

1 can of tomatoes

6oz quinoa

1 can chickpeas, drained

2 cups spinach

Directions:

Put the potatoes in a pan, covered in cold water and bring to the boil, then cook for 25 minutes they are soft (always check with a stick). Drain them well, remove the skin and put them a side.

Put garlic, turmeric, coriander, bean stew, ginger, coconut milk, tomato purée and tomatoes in a skillet. Bring to the boil, season with salt and pepper; at that point include the quinoa with an additional cup water.

Put on low heat, put a lid on and let simmer for 30 minutes, stirring occasionally. Halfway through cooking, put in the chickpeas. When there are only 5 minutes left, put in the spinach and potatoes, roughly chopped.

Split in 4 portions and serve immediately.

Nutrition Facts: Calories: 609 kcal Fat: 12.15 g Carbohydrates: 85.27 Protein: 23.04 g

Chili Sweetcorn And Wild Garlic Fritters

Preparation Time: 5 min

Cooking Time: 10 min

Servings: 4

Ingredients:

¾ cup Self-rising flour

2 cups Tinned or frozen sweetcorn

3 Medium free-range eggs

1 Red chili, finely chopped

Fry-light extra virgin olive oil spray

¾ cup Wild garlic leaves and bulbs, finely diced

2 cups lettuce, chopped

Direction:

Mix the eggs, flour, chili, diced wild garlic and sweetcorn in a bowl, season with the pepper and the salt.

Spray a large non-stick fry pan and put it on medium heat.

Use a spoon to scoop the egg mixture into the fry pan batch by batch. The mixture will give you two large fritters per person or four small fritters.

Fry the pancakes for about four minutes on one side, and then gently turn it to the other side and fry for another 3 min until it is set and golden brown.

Serve immediately with salad.

Nutrition Facts: Calories: 198 Fat: 7g Carbohydrates: 30g Protein: 3g

Roast Mackerel And Simple Veggies

Preparation Time: 5 min

Cooking Time: 25 min

Servings: 4

Ingredients:

2oz Pitted black olives

2 Leeks, chopped

7oz Cherry tomatoes

2 Sweet potatoes, chopped

1tbsp extra virgin olive oil

1 Lemon, juiced

11oz Mackerel fillets

¼ pint Vegetable stock

Directions:

Heat your oven to 375 degrees F. Place the chopped leeks and sweet potatoes in a roasting tray. Pour the vegetable stock over them and drizzle with the extra virgin oil.

Place the tray in the oven to roast for about 15 to 20 minutes.

Take out of the oven, add the black olives, cherry tomatoes, and mackerel fillets, and then squeeze the lemon juice all over. Return to the oven to roast other 10 minutes.

Serve immediately.

Nutrition Facts: Calories: 374 Fat: 12g Carbohydrate: 48g Protein: 17g

Baked Root Veg With Chili

Preparation Time: 20 minutes

Cooking Time: 50 minutes

Servings: 4

Ingredients:

3 medium Potatoes	2 stalks Celery
3 medium Sweet potatoes	2 medium Carrots
3 small Yam	1 Bell pepper
2 cups Vegetable broth	2 Red onions
1 can Red kidney beans	3 tbsp. Olive oil
1 can White kidney beans	½ oz. Cilantro
2 cans Diced tomatoes	2 Avocados
1 can Black beans	1 Bay leaf
1 tbsp. Dried oregano	1 can Sweet corn
2 tbsp. Paprika	2 Tomatoes
1 tsp Cumin	2 Limes, juiced
2 tsp Chili powder	1 head Romaine

Directions:

Scrub and fork the potatoes and yams. Drizzle them with oil. Sprinkle with salt and put on a baking tray for 45 minutes or until you can pierce easily with a knife.

Heat the oil in a frying pan on medium heat and add the diced onion with the chopped bell pepper, diced carrots, and celery along with a quarter tsp of salt.

Cook until the carrot is tender then add the paprika, oregano, cumin, and chili powder.

Put in tomato, the bay leaf, and the vegetable broth. Rinse the beans and drain well before adding to the pot.

Stir well and leave to simmer for a further 30 minutes. After this time has passed, get a potato masher and mash the chili a few times to crush part of the beans and thicken the mixture.

Add the juice of one lime, and salt and pepper to taste.

In a bowl, finely dice the avocado and lightly mash with salt, pepper and the juice of another lime.

In another bowl, drain and rinse the corn and toss in cilantro, finely chopped, shredded romaine lettuce a pinch of salt and a tbsp. olive oil.

Serve potatoes, chili, avocado and salad so that everyone can assemble his/her masterpiece. Enjoy!

Nutrition Facts: Calories: 493kcal; Fat: 14g; Carbohydrates: 96g Protein: 14g;

Autumn Stuffed Enchiladas

Preparation Time: 35 minutes

Cooking Time: 50 minutes

Servings: 2

Ingredients:

1 Lemon, juiced	2 tbsp. Olive oil
1 cup raw Cashews	¼ tbsp. Cayenne pepper
½ oz. Cilantro	1 tsp Chili flakes
1 oz. Roasted pumpkin seeds	1 tsp Cumin
12 Corn tortillas	3 cloves Garlic
2 cups Butternut squash	1 Jalapeno
1 cup Salsa	1 Red onion
1 can Black beans	1 cup Brussel sprouts

Directions:

Soak the cashews in boiling water and set aside.

Cut the squash in half and after scooping out the seeds; lightly rub olive oil. Sprinkle with a little salt and pepper before putting on a baking sheet face down. Cook for about forty-five minutes at 400F until it is cooked.

Heat one tbsp. olive oil in a pan on medium heat and put chopped onion in, stirring until soft. Finely dice the jalapeno and garlic and finely slice the Brussel sprouts. Add these three things to the fry pan and cook until the Brussels begin to wilt through.

Strain and rinse the black beans then add them to the fry pan and mix well.

When the squash is cooked and cool enough to handle, scrape out the soft insides away from the skin and put in a big bowl along with the Brussels mixture. Mix well again with salt and pepper to taste.

Put the tortillas in the oven to soften up (don't let them get crispy)

Spoon the squash mixture into the middle of the soft tortillas. Carefully roll them up to make little open-ended wraps, and then put in on baking tray with the open ends down to stop them from unrolling.

Do this for all twelve tortillas then pour the rest of the salsa on top and spread to coat evenly.

Change the temperature of the oven to 350F and bake for 30 minutes.

While these cooks put the drained, soaked cashews into a blender with one and a half cups cold water, lemon juice, and a quarter tsp salt.

Blend until smooth, adding water if it becomes too thick. This is your sour cream.

When enchiladas are done, leave to cool while you chop cilantro.

Then drizzle the sour cream generously over the dish and top with cilantro and pumpkin seeds.

Nutrition Facts: Calories: 333kcal; Fat: 11g Carbohydrate: 36g; Protein: 14g;

Creamy Vegetable Casserole

Preparation Time: 30 minutes

Cooking Time: 60 minutes

Servings: 2

Ingredients:

2 tbsp. Fresh rosemary	2 tbsp. Apple cider vinegar
1 tsp Dried basil	1 cup raw cashews
1tsp Dried oregano	2 Zucchini
3 cloves Garlic	1 stalk Broccoli
¼ cup Nutritional yeast	1 Cauliflower
2tbsp Olive oil	10 Russet potatoes

Directions:

Pour boiled water over the cashews and leave to soak. Cut up the cauliflower into small florets and boil until soft. When the cauliflower is done, drain it and put it in a blender along with the drained cashews and one and a half cups of cold water.

Add a good half tsp of salt along with the apple cider vinegar and nutritional yeast. Blend until creamy.

Wash and grate the zucchini, set aside. Cut the broccoli into small bite-sized pieces and set aside.

Spread the sides and bottom of a baking tray with olive oil. Cut the potatoes as thin as you can and spread them in the tray forming an even layer. Pour half of the cauliflower sauce to cover and spread evenly.

Add the grated zucchini and spread out to cover the sauce. Sprinkle the oregano and basil over the zucchini, then push the pieces of broccoli into the zucchini to keep the surface as even as possible.

Drizzle a little more cauliflower sauce around the broccoli pieces to fill in the gaps.

Do another layer to use up the rest of the potatoes, then pour the rest of the remaining cauliflower sauce over top of that.

Spread it out as evenly as possible, right to the edges to fill in all the gaps around the sides.

Sprinkle the top with a half tsp of black pepper and a generous pinch or two of salt. Finely chop the fresh rosemary and sprinkle that on top also.

Put in the oven on 400F for 45 minutes. It will be done when a knife pierces the potatoes without pulling them up and the top should be beautifully browned. Let it cool before serving.

Nutrition Facts: Calories: 389kcal; Fat: 4g; Carbohydrate: 37g; Protein: 26g

Vegan Mac And Cheese

Preparation Time: 25 minutes

Cooking Time: 30 minutes

Servings: 2

Ingredients:

1 cup raw Cashews	3 cloves Garlic
½ tsp Chili flakes	1 Russet potato
½ cup Nutritional yeast	1 White onion
Salt and pepper to taste	2tbsp Avocado oil
½ tsp mustard powder	1 head Broccoli
½ tsp Onion powder	1 ½ tsp Apple cider vinegar
½ tsp Garlic powder	2 cups Macaroni

Directions:

Peel and grate the potato. Finely dice the garlic. Heat a large saucepan and oil over medium heat. Put onion and a little salt in the pot and cook until soft.

Add potato, chili flakes, garlic, mustard, onion and garlic powders into the pot. Stir well until their flavors release, then add one cup of water and cashews. Keep stirring at a simmer until the potatoes are soft.

Pour entire mixture into a blender along with the apple cider vinegar and nutritional yeast, salt and pepper. The consistency should be that of cheese sauce that is thick yet runny. If it is too thick, add more water, if it needs more salt or garlic powder, chili flakes or vinegar, do so now according to your taste.

Boil the pasta in salted water. In another pot, boil the broccoli in bite-sized florets until tender. When both are ready, transfer everything into one pot and cover with the cheese sauce. Combine well, serve and enjoy!

Nutrition Facts: Calories: 263kcal; Fat: 14g; carbohydrates: 36g; Protein: 4g;

Butternut Squash Alfredo

Preparation Time: 15 minutes

Cooking Time: 25 minutes

Servings: 4

Ingredients:

9oz Whole grain linguine	1 White onion
2 cups Vegetable broth	1 cup Green peas
3 cups Butternut Squash, diced	1 Zucchini
Salt and pepper to taste	2tbsp Olive oil
1 tsp Paprika	2 tbsp. Sage
2 cloves Garlic	

Directions:

Heat the oil in a large fry pan with medium heat. While it heats, ensures the sage leaves are clean and dry, then them put in the oil to fry, moving around not to burn.

Pull them out and put them on a paper towel.

Into the fry pan, put the peeled and diced squash along with paprika, diced onion, and black pepper.

Cook until the onion is soft then add the broth and salt to taste.

Bring to a boil before turning down to low heat and leaving the squash to cook through. In another pot, cook the linguine in water with a little salt.

When the squash is tender, put it in a blender along with all the liquid and other ingredients. Blend until creamy and taste to see if more salt, pepper or spice is needed.

Put it back in the fry pan to keep warm on low heat.

Using a grater, grate the zucchini lengthwise to make long noodles. Make as many long ones as you can to blend in with the linguine.

Add them to the sauce along with the green peas and cook in the butternut squash for five minutes.

When the pasta is done, save one cup of liquid before you drain it. Add the linguine to the pasta and stir well to coat the linguine.

If the sauce is too thick, add a little of pasta water. Serve the pasta topped with the fried sage leaves and a little blacker pepper.

Nutrition Facts: Calories: 432; Fat: 14g; Carbohydrate: 36g; Protein: 34g;

Vegan Lasagna

Preparation Time: 25 minutes

Cooking Time: 60 minutes

Servings: 2

Ingredients:

4 tbsp. tapioca starch

¼ tsp salt

1 tbsp. Apple cider vinegar

4 medium lemons, juiced

1 cup raw cashews

3 cups Baby spinach

1 box Lasagna noodles

2 Zucchini

½ tsp Garlic powder

2 tsp Dried oregano

2 tsp Dried basil

Salt and pepper to taste

2 tbsp. Olive oil

½ cup Nutritional yeast

16 oz. firm tofu

3 tbsp. Tomato puree

1 tbsp. onion powder

6 cloves of garlic

1 medium white onion

Salt and pepper

2 cans crushed tomatoes

1 cup red lentils, drained

Directions:

Put three cups of water in a saucepan with the lentils, then bring to a boil before reducing to a simmer for around twenty minutes. Drain the lentils and set aside.

In the same saucepan, add oil and the diced onion and let it cool down.

When the onion is soft, add finely diced garlic, generous pinches of salt and pepper, and one tsp of dried oregano and basil, the two cans of tomato and the tomato puree. Leave to simmer for 15 minutes, stirring every 5 minutes.

Add the lentils to this then set aside. This is the marinara sauce.

Put one cup of cashews into a bowl with two cups of boiled water and set aside.

Wash and slice the zucchini into lengthwise strips that are long and relatively thin then set aside.

Break up the tofu and add to the blender along with the juice from one lemon, one tsp each of basil and oregano, the nutritional yeast, garlic powder, and a little salt.

Keep pulsing until it is mostly smooth but still a little textured. Put into a bowl and set aside, this is your ricotta.

Drain the soaked cashews and put them into a clean blender with the apple cider vinegar, the juice from one lemon, tapioca starch, and a little salt. Pour in one and a half cups of water and blend until smooth.

Pour this into a saucepan on medium heat and stir until it becomes stretchy then set aside. This is the cheese sauce.

In a large baking dish, place a few spoonsful of the marinara sauce and spread it to cover the bottom and sides of the dish. Begin to layer the lasagna noodles, the ricotta, the zucchini, and the cheese sauce. Follow this with half of the spinach, more marinara, lasagna noodles, spinach, and the cheese sauce. Keep repeating until all ingredients have been used except for a small portion of the cheese sauce.

Put into a 350F oven for 45 minutes on the highest shelf. Remove after 40 minutes and spoon the remainder of the cheese sauce over the top to resemble mozzarella blobs, then return to the oven for 5 to 10 more minutes. Let rest then serve and enjoy!

Nutrition Facts: Calories: 543kcal; Fat: 14g; Carbohydrate: 76g; Protein: 34g

Cajun Turkey Rice

Preparation Time: 10 minutes

Cooking Time: 25 minutes

Servings: 4

Ingredients:

5 quarts chicken broth

2 cups uncooked white rice

1 ½ cups celery, chopped

1 ½ cups red onion, chopped

1 tbsp. garlic, minced

8oz ground pork

8oz ground beef

2 tbsp. Cajun seasoning

1 tbsp. dried thyme

1 tbsp. dried parsley

1 tbsp. dried oregano

Directions:

Place the chicken broth, rice, celery, and 1 cup of chopped onion into a large pot. Bring to a boil over high heat. Reduce heat to medium-low, cover, and simmer until the rice is tender, 20 to 25 minutes.

Meanwhile, place the remaining ½ cup of onion into a large skillet along with the garlic, pork, and beef.

Cook and stir over medium-high heat until the meat is brown and crumbly. Pour off excess grease, and then stir the meat into the cooked rice along with the thyme, parsley, and oregano.

Stir well and serve.

Nutrition Facts: Calories: 134 Carbs: 27g Fat: 2g Protein: 4g

Tomato & Goat's Cheese Pizza

Preparation Time: 5 Minutes

Cooking Time: 50 Minutes

Servings: 2

Ingredients:

8oz buckwheat flour

2 teaspoons dried yeast

Pinch of salt

5fl oz. slightly water

1 tsp olive oil

3oz feta cheese, crumbled

3ozpassata or tomato paste

1 tomato, sliced

1 red onion, finely chopped

1oz rocket arugula leaves, chopped

Directions:

In a bowl, combine all the ingredients for the pizza dough then allow it to stand for at least an hour until it has doubled in size.

Roll the dough out to a size to suit you. Spoon the passata onto the base and add the rest of the toppings. Bake in the oven at 400F for 15-20 minutes or until browned at the edges and crispy and serve.

Nutrition Facts: Calories 387 kcal, Fat 9.9g, Carbohydrate 52g, Protein 8.4g

Side Dishes

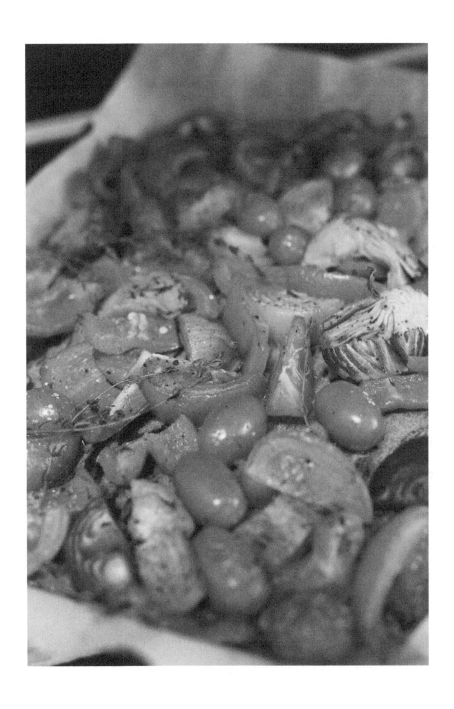

Sage Carrots

Preparation Time: 10 minutes

Cooking Time: 25 minutes

Servings: 2

Ingredients:

2 tsps. Sweet paprika

1 tbsp. chopped sage

2 tbsps. Olive oil

1 lb. peeled and roughly cubed carrots

¼ tsp. black pepper

1 chopped red onion

Directions:

In a baking pan, combine the carrots with the oil and the other ingredients, toss and bake at 380 0F for 30 minutes. Divide between plates and serve.

Nutrition Facts: Calories: 200 kcal, Fat: 8.7 g, Carbs: 7.9 g, Protein: 4 g,

Pesto Green Beans

Preparation Time: 10 minutes

Cooking Time: 55 minutes

Servings: 2

Ingredients:

2 tbsps. Olive oil

2 tsps. Sweet paprika

Juice of 1 lemon

2 tbsp. Basil pesto

1 lb. trimmed and halved green beans

¼ tsp. black pepper

1 sliced red onion

Directions:

Heat up a pan with the oil over medium-high heat; add the onion, stir and sauté for 5 minutes. Add the beans and the rest of the ingredients, toss, cook over medium heat for 10 minutes, divide between plates and serve.

Nutrition Facts: Calories: 280 kcal, Fat: 10 g, Carbs: 13.9 g, Protein: 4.7 g,

Minty Tomatoes and Corn

Preparation Time: 10 minutes

Cooking Time: 65 minutes

Servings: 2

Ingredients:

2 cups corn

1 tbsp. rosemary vinegar

2 tbsp. Chopped mint

1 lb. sliced tomatoes

¼ tsp. black pepper

2 tbsp. Olive oil

Directions: In a salad bowl, combine the tomatoes with the corn and the other ingredients, toss and serve. Enjoy!

Nutrition Facts: Calories: 230 kcal, Fat: 7.2 g, Carbs: 11.6 g, Protein: 4 g

Roasted Beets

Preparation Time: 10 minutes

Cooking Time: 40 minutes

Servings: 2

Ingredients:

2 minced garlic cloves

¼ tsp black pepper

4 peeled and sliced beets

¼ cup chopped walnuts

2 tbsp. Olive oil

¼ cup chopped parsley

Directions:

In a baking dish, combine the beets with the oil and the other ingredients, toss to coat, put in the oven at 420°F, and bake for 30 minutes.

Divide between plates and serve.

Nutrition Facts: Calories: 156 kcal, Fat: 11.8 g, Carbs: 11.5 g, Protein: 3.8 g

Kale Sauté

Preparation Time: 10 minutes

Cooking Time: 15 minutes

Servings: 2

Ingredients:

- 1 chopped red onion
- 3 tbsp. Coconut aminos
- 2 tbsp. Olive oil
- 1 lb. torn kale

- 1 tbsp. chopped cilantro
- 1 tbsp. lime juice
- 2 minced garlic cloves

Directions:

Heat up a pan with the olive oil over medium heat; add the onion and the garlic and sauté for 5 minutes.

Add the kale and the other ingredients, toss, cook over medium heat for 10 minutes, divide between plates and serve.

Nutrition Facts: Calories: 200 kcal, Fat: 7.1 g, Carbs: 6.4 g, Protein: 6 g

Rosemary Endives

Preparation Time: 10 minutes

Cooking Time: 20 minutes

Servings: 2

Ingredients:

2 tbsp. Olive oil

1 tsp. dried rosemary

2 halved endives

¼ tsp. black pepper

½ tsp. turmeric powder

Directions:

In a baking pan, combine the endives with the oil and the other ingredients, toss gently, introduce in the oven and bake at 400 0F for 20 minutes. Divide between plates and serve.

Nutrition Facts: Calories: 66 kcal, Fat: 7.1 g, Carbs: 1.2 g, Protein: 0.3 g

Scallops with Almonds and Mushrooms

Preparation Time: 5 minutes

Cooking Time: 10 minutes

Servings: 4

Ingredients:

1-pound scallops

2 tbsp. olive oil

4 scallions, chopped

½ cup mushrooms, sliced

2 tbsp. almonds, chopped

1 cup coconut cream

Directions:

Heat up a pan with the oil over medium heat; add the scallions and the mushrooms and sauté for 2 minutes.

Add the scallops cook over medium heat for 8 minutes more, divide into bowls and serve.

Nutrition Facts: Calories 322 kcal, Fat 23.7g, Carbohydrate 8.1g, Protein 21.6g

Thyme Mushrooms

Preparation Time: 10 minutes

Cooking Time: 30 minutes

Servings: 2

Ingredients:

1 tbsp. chopped thyme

2 tbsp. Olive oil

2 tbsp. Chopped parsley

4 minced garlic cloves

Salt and Black pepper to taste

2 lbs. halved white mushrooms

Directions:

In a baking pan, combine the mushrooms with the garlic and the other ingredients, toss, introduce in the oven and cook at 400°F for 30 minutes.

Divide between plates and serve.

Nutrition Facts: Calories: 251kcal, Fat: 9.3 g, Carbs: 13.2 g, Protein: 6 g

Apples and Cabbage Mix

Preparation Time: 10 minutes

Cooking Time:

Servings: 4

Ingredients:

2 cored and cubed green apples

2 tbsp. Balsamic vinegar

½ tsp. caraway seeds

2 tbsp. Olive oil

Black pepper

1 shredded red cabbage head

Directions:

In a bowl, combine the cabbage with the apples and the other ingredients, toss and serve.

Nutrition Facts: Calories: 165 kcal, Fat: 7.4 g, Carbs: 26 g, Protein: 2.6 g

Carrot, Tomato, And Arugula Quinoa Pilaf

Preparation Time: 10 minutes

Cooking Time: 35 minutes

Servings: 4

Ingredients:

2 teaspoons extra virgin olive oil

½ red onion, chopped

1 cup quinoa, raw

2 cups vegetable or chicken broth

1 tsp fresh lovage, chopped

1 carrot, chopped

1 tomato, chopped

1 cup baby arugula

Directions:

Heat the olive oil in a saucepan over medium heat and add the red onion. Cook and stir until translucent, about 5 minutes.

Lower the heat, stir in quinoa, and toast, stirring constantly, for 2 minutes. Stir in the broth, black pepper, and thyme.

Raise the heat to high and bring to a boil. Cover, reduce heat to low, and simmer for 5 minutes.

Stir in the carrots, cover and simmer until all water is absorbed, about 10 more minutes.

Turn off the heat, add tomatoes, arugula and lovage and let sit for 5 minutes. Add salt and pepper to taste.

Nutrition Facts: Calories: 165 kcal Fat: 4g Carbs: 27g Protein: 6g

Bake Kale Walnut

Preparation Time: 10 minutes

Cooking Time: 30 minutes

Servings: 4

Ingredients

1 medium red onion, finely chopped

¼ cup extra virgin olive oil

2 cups baby kale

½ cup half-and-half cream

½ cup walnuts, coarsely chopped

1/3 cup dry breadcrumbs

½ tsp ground nutmeg

Salt and pepper to taste

¼ cup dry breadcrumbs

2 tbsp. extra virgin olive oil

Directions

Preheat oven to 350 degrees F. In a skillet, sauté onion in olive oil until tender. In a large bowl, combine cooked onion, kale, cream, walnuts, breadcrumbs, nutmeg and salt and pepper to taste, mixing well.

Transfer to a greased 1-1/2-qt. baking dish. Combine topping ingredients and sprinkle over the kale mixture. Bake, uncovered, for 30 minutes or until lightly browned.

Nutrition Facts: Calories: 555 Fat: 31g Carbs: 65g Protein: 26g

Arugula With Apples And Pine Nuts

Preparation Time: 10 minutes

Cooking Time: 8 minutes

Servings: 4

Ingredients:

2 tbsp. extra virgin olive oil

2 cloves garlic, slivered

2 tbsp. pine nuts

1 apple, peeled, cored and chopped

10 oz. arugula

Salt and pepper to taste

Directions:

Heat the olive oil in a large skillet or wok over low heat. Add the garlic, pine nuts, and apple. Cook until the nuts and garlic are golden, and the apple is just starting to soften, 3 to 5 minutes. Increase the heat to medium and add the arugula. Stir and cook another 2 to 3 minutes. Season with salt and pepper to taste.

Nutrition Facts: Calories: 121 Fat: 9g Carbs: 8g Protein: 3g

Kale Green Bean Casserole

Preparation Time: 5 minutes

Cooking Time: 40 minutes

Servings: 4

Ingredients:

1 ½ cups milk

1 cup sour cream

1 cup mushrooms, chopped

2 cups green beans, chopped

2 cups kale, chopped

¼ cup capers, drained

¼ cup walnuts, crushed

Directions:

Preheat the oven to 375 degrees F and lightly grease a casserole dish.

Whisk the milk and sour cream together in a large bowl.

Add mushrooms, green beans, kale, and capers. Pour into the casserole dish and top with the crushed walnuts.

Bake uncovered in the preheated oven until bubbly and browned on top, about 40 minutes.

Nutrition Facts: Calories: 130 Fat: 6g Carbs: 14g Protein: 2g

Rice With Lemon And Arugula

Preparation Time: 10 minutes

Cooking Time: 35 minutes

Servings: 4

Ingredients:

1 small red onion, chopped

1 cup fresh mushrooms, sliced

2 cloves garlic, minced

1 tbsp. extra-virgin olive oil

3 cups long-grain rice, steamed

10 oz. fresh arugula

3 tbsp. lemon juice

¼ tsp dill weed

Salt and pepper to taste

1/3 cup feta cheese, crumbled

Directions:

Pre-heat and oven to 350°F. In a skillet, sauté the onion, mushrooms and garlic in oil until tender. Stir in the rice, arugula, lemon juice, dill and salt and pepper to taste.

Reserve 1 tbsp. cheese and stir the rest into skillet; mix well. Transfer to an 8-in. square baking dish coated with nonstick cooking spray. Sprinkle with reserved cheese. Cover and bake for 25 minutes.

Uncover and bake for an additional 5-10 minutes or until heated through and cheese is melted.

Nutrition Facts: Calories 290kcal, Fat 6g, Carbohydrate 55g, Protein 13g

Easy Cajun Grilled Veggies

Preparation Time: 50 minutes

Cooking Time: 5 minutes

Servings: 4

Ingredients:

¼ cup extra virgin olive oil

1 tsp Cajun seasoning

1/2 tsp cayenne pepper

1 tbsp. Worcestershire sauce

2 zucchinis cut into 1/2-inch slices

2 large red onions, sliced into ½" wedges

2 yellow squash, cut into 1/2-inch slices

Directions:

In a small bowl, mix together olive oil, Cajun seasoning, cayenne pepper, and Worcestershire sauce. Place zucchinis, onions, and yellow squash in a bowl, and cover with the olive oil mixture. Salt to taste.

Cover bowl and marinate vegetables in the refrigerator at least 30 minutes. Preheat an outdoor grill for high heat and lightly oil grate. Place marinated vegetable pieces on skewers or directly on the grill. Cook 5 minutes until done.

Nutrition Facts: Calories: 95kcal, Fat: 7g Carbs: 8g, Protein: 2g

Purple Potatoes With Onions, Mushrooms And Capers

Preparation Time: 10 minutes

Cooking Time: 25 minutes

Servings: 4

Ingredients:

6 purple potatoes, scrubbed

3 tbsp. extra virgin olive oil

1 large red onion, chopped

8 oz. fresh mushrooms, sliced

Salt and pepper to taste

¼ tsp chili pepper flakes

1 tbsp. capers, drained and chopped

1 tsp fresh tarragon, chopped

Directions:

Cut each potato into wedges by quartering the potatoes, then cutting each quarter in half. Heat 1 tbsp. of olive oil over medium heat in a large skillet and cook the onion and mushrooms until the mushrooms start to release their liquid and the onion becomes translucent, about 5 minutes. Transfer the onion and mushrooms into a bowl and set aside.

Heat 2 more tbsp. of olive oil over high heat in the same skillet and add the potato wedges into the hot oil. Sprinkle with salt and pepper, and allow to cook, stirring occasionally, until the wedges are browned on both sides, about 10 minutes.

Reduce heat to medium, sprinkle the potato wedges with red pepper flakes, and allow to cook until the potatoes are tender, about 10 more minutes. Stir in the onion and mushroom mixture, toss the vegetables together, and mix in the capers and fresh tarragon.

Nutrition Facts: Calories: 215 Fat: 6g Carbs: 23g Protein: 3g

Vegetarian Stuffed Peppers

Preparation Time: 10 minutes

Cooking Time: 70 minutes

Servings: 6

Ingredients:

1 ½ cups brown rice, uncooked

6 large green bell peppers

3 tbsp. soy sauce

3 tbsp. dry red wine

1 tsp vegetarian Worcestershire sauce

1 ½ cups extra firm tofu

1/2 cup sweetened dried cranberries

¼ cup walnuts, chopped

½ cup Parmesan, grated

Salt and pepper, to taste

2 cups tomato sauce

2 tbsp. brown sugar

Directions:

Preheat oven to 350°F. In a saucepan bring 3 cups water to a boil. Stir in rice. Reduce heat, cover and simmer for 40 minutes. Meanwhile, core and seed green peppers, leaving bottoms intact.

Place peppers in a microwavable dish with about ½" of water in the bottom. Microwave on high for 6 minutes. In a small saucepan, bring soy sauce, wine and Worcestershire sauce to a simmer. Add tofu and simmer until the liquid is absorbed.

Combine rice, tofu, cranberries, nuts, cheese, salt and pepper in a large bowl and mix well. Pack rice firmly into peppers. Return peppers to the dish you first microwaved them in and bake for 25 to 30 minutes, or until lightly browned on top.

Meanwhile, in a small saucepan over low heat, combine tomato sauce and brown sugar. Heat until hot.

Serve stuffed peppers with the tomato sauce spooned over each serving.

Nutrition Facts: Calories: 250 Carbs: 22g Fat: 10g Protein: 17g

Roasted Red Endive With Caper Butter

Preparation Time: 10 minutes

Cooking Time: 25 minutes

Servings: 4

Ingredients:

10 red endives

2 tsp. extra virgin olive oil

2 anchovy fillets, packed in oil

1 small lemon, juiced

3 tbsp. capers, drained

5 tbsp. cold butter, cut into cubes

1 tbsp. fresh parsley, chopped

Salt and pepper as needed

Directions:

Preheat the oven to 425°F. Toss endives with olive oil, salt, and pepper, and spread out on to a baking sheet cut side down.

Bake for about 20-25 minutes or until caramelized.

While they're roasting, add the anchovies to a large pan over medium heat and use a fork to mash them until broken up.

 Add lemon juice and mix well, then add capers.

Lower the heat and slowly stir in the butter and parsley. Drizzle butter over roasted endives, season as necessary and garnish with more fresh parsley.

Nutrition Facts: calories 109 fat 8.6g protein1.5 g, carbohydrates 4.9 g, Fiber 4 g

Chickpeas With Caramelized Onion And Endive

Preparation Time: 10 minutes

Cooking Time: 25 minutes

Servings: 4

Ingredients:

2 large red endives

¼ cup extra-virgin olive oil

2 medium red onions, sliced thinly

2 tsp sugar

¼ cup Medjool dates, chopped

Salt and pepper, to taste

2 cans of chickpeas

Directions:

Prepare the endives discarding the external leaves and the core. Wash them in a large bowl of cold water then cut them into large pieces and set aside.

Heat the oil over medium heat in a large skillet.

Add the onions and cook until translucent, about 5 minutes. Stir in the sugar, and continue cooking until the onions are golden brown, about 10 minutes.

Add the dates and the endive leaves.

Cook, stirring occasionally, until the leaves are tender, about 6 minutes. Season with salt and pepper to taste.

Stir in the chickpeas and let cook until the flavors have blended, for about 5 minutes.

Nutrition Facts: Calories: 288 Fat: 6g Carbohydrate: 52g Protein: 10g

Sauces and dressings

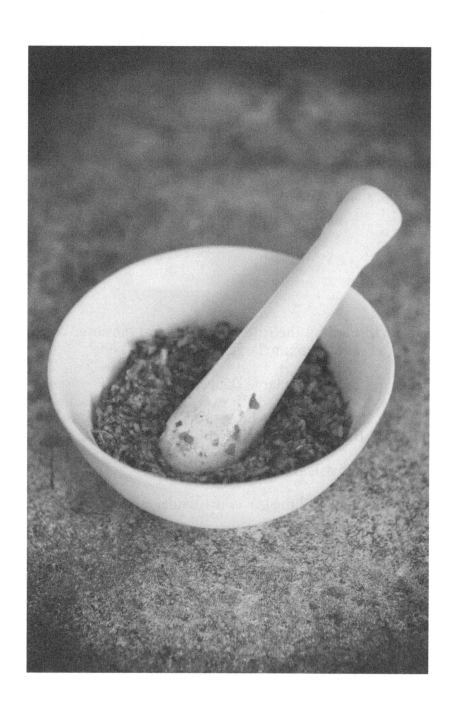

Salsa Verde

Preparation Time: 20 minutes

Cooking Time: 10minutes

Servings: 4

Ingredients:

½ cup fresh parsley, finely chopped

3 tbsp. fresh basil, finely chopped

2 cloves garlic, crushed

¾ cup olive oil

2 tbsp. small capers

½ lemon, the juice

½ tsp ground black pepper

1 tsp sea salt

Directions:

Add all of the ingredients to a deep bowl and mix with an immersion blender until the sauce has the desired consistency.

Store the sauce in the refrigerator for up to 4-5 days or in the freezer.

Nutrition Facts: Calories 323, Fat 37g, Carbohydrates 2g, Protein 1g

Tzatziki

Preparation Time: 30 minutes

Cooking Time: 0 minutes

Servings: 6

Ingredients:

½ cucumber

1 cup Greek yogurt

1 tbsp. olive oil

2 cloves garlic

1 tbsp. fresh mint, finely chopped

Pinch of ground black pepper

1 tsp salt

Directions:

Rinse the cucumber grate it with a grater without peeling it. The green skin adds color and texture to the sauce.

Put the grated cucumber in a strainer and sprinkle salt on top. Mix well and let the liquid drain for 5-10 minutes. Wrap cucumber in a tea towel and squeeze out excess liquid.

Crush garlic and place it in a bowl. Add cucumber, oil and fresh mint.

Stir in the yogurt and add black pepper and salt to taste. Let the sauce sit in the refrigerator for at least 10 minutes for the flavors to develop.

Nutrition Facts: Calories 81, Fat 7g, Carbohydrates 3g, Protein 1g

Guacamole

Preparation Time: 15 minutes

Cooking Time: 0 minutes

Servings: 4

Ingredients:

2 ripe avocados

1 clove garlic

3 tbsp. olive oil

½ white onion

1 tomato, diced

5 1/3 tbsp. fresh cilantro

½ lime, the juice

Salt and pepper

Directions:

Peel the avocados and mash with a fork. Grate or chop the onion finely and add to the mash. Squeeze the lime and add the juice.

Add tomato, olive oil and finely chopped cilantro. Season with salt and pepper and mix well.

Let the sauce sit in the refrigerator for at least 10 minutes for the flavors to develop.

Nutrition Facts: Calories 244, Fat 25g, Carbohydrates 5g, Protein 3g

Avocado Caesar Dressing

Preparation Time: 10 minutes

Cooking Time: 0 minutes

Servings: 4

Ingredients:

1/3 cup avocado, mashed

2 cloves garlic, minced

1 tbsp. olive oil

2 anchovy fillets or 1 tsp anchovy paste

3 tbsp. lemon juice

¼ cup Parmesan cheese, shredded

2 tbsp. almond milk, unsweetened

2 teaspoons Worcestershire sauce

½ tsp mustard

2 tbsp. water

¾ tsp sea salt

¼ tsp ground pepper

Directions:

Add all ingredients into a high-powered blender or food processor and blend until smooth.

Taste and add additional salt and pepper if needed.

Nutrition Facts: Calories 58, Fat 5g, Carbohydrates 2g, Protein 2g

Italian Veggie Salsa

Preparation Time: 10 minutes

Cooking Time: 10 minutes

Servings: 4

Ingredients:

2 red bell peppers cut into wedges

3 zucchinis, sliced

½ cup garlic, minced

2 tbsp. olive oil

A pinch of black pepper

1 tsp Italian seasoning

Directions:

Heat up a pan with the oil over medium-high heat, add bell peppers and zucchini, toss and cook for 5 minutes.

Add garlic, black pepper and Italian seasoning, toss, cook for 5 minutes more.

Blitz in a food processor when done until completely smooth.

Nutrition Facts: Calories 132 kcal, Fat 3g, Carbohydrate 7g, Protein 4g

Black Bean Salsa

Preparation Time: 10 minutes

Cooking Time: 0 minutes

Servings: 6

Ingredients:

1 tbsp. coconut aminos

½ tsp cumin, ground

1 cup canned black beans, drained

1 cup salsa

6 cups romaine lettuce leaves, torn

½ cup avocado, pitted and cubed

Directions:

In a bowl, combine the beans with the aminos, cumin, salsa, lettuce and avocado, toss, divide into small bowls and serve as a snack.

Nutrition Facts: Calories 181 kcal, Fat 4g, Carbohydrate 14g, Protein 7g

Mung Sprouts Salsa

Preparation Time: 10 minutes

Cooking Time: 0 minutes

Servings: 2

Ingredients:

1 red onion, chopped

2 cups mung beans, sprouted

A pinch of red chili powder

1 green chili pepper, chopped

1 tomato, chopped

1 tsp chaat masala

1 tsp lemon juice

1 tbsp. coriander, chopped

Directions:

In a salad bowl, mix onion with mung sprouts, chili pepper, tomato, chili powder, chaat masala, lemon juice, coriander and pepper, toss well, divide into small cups and serve.

Nutrition Facts: Calories 100 kcal, Fat 2g, Carbohydrate 3g, Protein 6g

Jerusalem Artichoke Gratin

Preparation Time: 10 minutes

Cooking Time: 45 minutes

Servings: 3

Ingredients:

1lb Jerusalem artichoke

1 cup milk

3tbsp grated cheese

1 tbsp. crème Fraiche

1tsp butter

Curry, paprika powder, nutmeg, salt, pepper

Directions:

Wash and peel the Jerusalem artichokes and slice them into approx. ½ inch thick slices. Bring them to a boil with the milk in a saucepan. Then stir in the spices and crème Fraiche.

Grease a baking dish with butter and add the Jerusalem artichoke and milk mixture. Bake on the middle shelf in the oven for about half an hour at 325°F..

Sprinkle with grated cheese and bake five minutes before the end of the baking time.

Nutrition Facts: Calories: 133 Net carbs: 9.9g Fat: 8.1g Fiber: 1.1g Protein: 4.7g

Salads

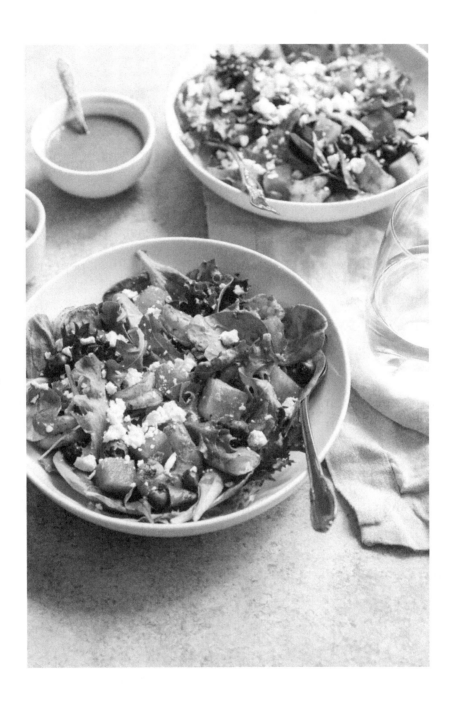

Greek Salad Skewers

Preparation Time: 10 minutes

Cooking Time: 0 minutes

Servings: 2

Ingredients:

8 big black olives

8 cherry tomatoes

1 yellow pepper, cut into 8 squares

½ red onion, split into 8 wedges

1 cucumber, cut into 8 pieces

4 oz. feta, cut into 8 cubes

1 tbsp. extra-virgin olive oil

Juice of 1/2 lemon

1 tsp balsamic vinegar

1/2 teaspoons garlic, crushed

Ground Black pepper

Salt

Directions:

Put the salad ingredients on the skewers following this order: cherry tomato, yellow pepper, red onion, cucumber, feta, black olive.

Repeat for each skewer and put on a serving plate.

As dressing, put in a small bowl: olive oil, a pinch of salt and pepper, lemon juice, balsamic vinegar and crushed garlic. Whisk well and drizzle on the skewers.

Nutrition Facts: Calories: 236kcal Fat: 21g Carbohydrate: 14g Protein: 7g

Sesame Chicken Salad

Preparation Time: 12 minutes

Cooking Time: 0 minutes

Servings: 2

Ingredients:

1 tbsp. sesame seeds

1 cucumber, chopped

4 oz. baby spinach, roughly sliced

2 oz. pak choi, really finely chopped

1/2 red onion, very finely chopped

6 oz. cooked chicken, shredded

For the dressing:

1 tbsp. extra-virgin olive oil

1 tsp sesame oil

Juice of 1 lime

1 tsp clear honey

2 tsp soy sauce

Directions:

Toast the sesame seeds in a dry skillet for two minutes till lightly browned and aromatic. Transfer to a plate to cool. In a bowl mix together the olive oil, sesame oil, lime juice, honey and soy sauce to create the dressing.

Put the cucumber, peeled, halved lengthways, deseeded using a teaspoon and chopped in a large bowl. Add spinach, pak choi, red onion and mix. Pour on the dressing and mix.

Divide the salad between 2 plates and top with the shredded chicken. Distribute on the sesame seeds just before serving.

Nutrition Facts: Calories: 391 Fat: 15g Carbohydrate: 20g Protein: 39g

Coronation Chicken Salad

Preparation Time: 15 minutes

Cooking Time: 0 minutes

Servings: 1

Ingredients:

3 oz. Natural yoghurt

Juice of 1/4 of a lemon

1 tsp Coriander, chopped

1 tsp Ground turmeric

1/2 tsp. moderate curry powder

4 oz. Cooked chicken breast

6 Walnut halves, finely chopped

2 Medjool dates, thinly sliced

20 grams Red onion, diced

1 Bird's eye chili

1 oz. Rocket

Direction:

Cut the chicken breast to bite-sized pieces

In a serving plate put the rocket as a base, then sprinkle the chicken, walnuts, dates, onion.

Mix yoghurt, lemon juice, spices and coriander together in a small bowl and drizzle it over the salad.

Nutrition Facts: Calories: 364 Fat: 12g Carbohydrate: 45g Protein: 15g

Sirt Fruit Salad

Preparation Time: 10 minutes

Cooking Time: 0 minutes

Servings: 1

Ingredients:

1/2 cup freshly produced green tea

1 tsp honey

1 orange, halved

1 apple, cored and roughly chopped

10 red seedless grapes

10 blueberries

Directions:

Stir the honey into half a cup of green tea and let it chill.

When chilled, add the juice of half orange.

Slice the other half and put in a bowl with the chopped apple, blueberries and grapes.

Pour over the tea and let rest in the fridge for 30 minutes before serving.

Nutrition Facts: Calories: 110 Fat: 0g Carbohydrate: 17g Protein: 2g.

Fresh Salad With Orange Dressing

Preparation Time: 10 minutes

Cooking Time: 0 minutes

Servings: 2

Ingredients:

½ cup lettuce

1 medium yellow bell pepper

1 medium Red pepper

4 oz. Carrot, grated

10 Almonds

Ingredients dressing:

4 tbsp. Olive oil

½ cup Orange juice

1 tbsp. Apple cider vinegar

Salt and pepper to taste

Direction:

Clean the peppers and cut them into long thin strips. Tear off the lettuce leaves and cut them into smaller pieces.

Mix the salad with the peppers and the carrots in a bowl. Roughly chop the almonds and sprinkle over the salad.

Mix all the ingredients for the dressing in a bowl. Pour the dressing over the salad just before serving.

Nutrition Facts: Calories: 150 Fat: 10g Carbohydrate: 11g Protein: 2g

Tomato And Avocado Salad

Preparation Time: 10 minutes

Cooking Time: 0 minutes

Servings: 1

Ingredients:

1 large Tomato

4 oz. Cherry tomatoes

1/2 medium Red onion

1 ripe Avocado

1tsp fresh oregano

1tbsp. extra virgin olive oil

1 tsp White wine vinegar

1 pinch Celtic sea salt

Direction:

Cut the tomato into thick slices. Cut half of the cherry tomatoes into slices and the other half in half. Cut the red onion into super thin half rings. (if you have it, use a mandolin for this)

Cut the avocado into 6 parts. Spread the tomatoes on a plate, place the avocado on top.

Sprinkle red onion and oregano and drizzle olive oil, vinegar and a pinch of salt on the salad.

Nutrition Facts: Calories: 165 Fat: 14g Carbohydrate: 7g Protein: 5g

Arugula With Fruits And Nuts

Preparation Time: 10 minutes

Cooking Time: 3 minutes

Servings: 1

Ingredients:

½ cup Arugula

1 Peach

1/2 medium Red onion

¼ cup Blueberries

5 Pecans

Ingredients dressing:

1/2 medium Peach

1 tbsp. Olive oil

2 tbsp. White wine vinegar

1 sprig fresh basil

Directions:

Halve the peach and remove the seed.

Heat a grill pan and grill it briefly on both sides. Cut the red onion into thin half rings. Roughly chop the pecans.

Heat a pan and roast the pecans in it until they are fragrant.

Place the arugula on a plate and spread peaches, red onions, blueberries and roasted pecans over it.

Put all the ingredients for the dressing in a food processor and mix to an even dressing. Drizzle the dressing over the salad.

Nutrition Facts: Calories: 160 Fat: 7g Carbohydrate: 25g Protein: 3g

Spinach Salad With Asparagus And Salmon

Preparation Time: 20 minutes

Cooking Time: 8 minutes

Servings: 1

Ingredients:

2 cups Spinach

2 Eggs

4 oz. smoked salmon

1 cup Asparagus tips

4 oz. Cherry tomatoes

Lemon 1/2 pieces

1 tsp Olive oil

Directions:

Boil the eggs until they are done (6 minutes for soft boiled, 8 minutes for hard boiled). Heat a pan with a little oil and fry the asparagus tips . Halve cherry tomatoes.

Place the spinach on a plate and spread the asparagus tips, cherry tomatoes and smoked salmon on top.

Peel and halve the eggs. Add them to the salad. Squeeze the lemon and drizzle some olive oil over it.

Season the salad with a little salt and pepper.

Nutrition Facts: Calories: 552 Fat: 40g Carbohydrate: 6g Protein: 39g

Brunoise Salad

Preparation Time: 10 minutes

Cooking Time: 0 minutes

Servings: 1

Ingredients:

1 large tomato

1 medium zucchini

1/2 medium red bell pepper

1/2 medium yellow bell pepper

1/2 medium red onion

3 springs fresh parsley

1/2 Lemon

2 tbsp. Olive oil

Directions:

Finely dice tomatoes, zucchini, peppers and red onions to get a brunoise. Mix all the cubes in a bowl. Chop parsley and mix in the salad. Squeeze the lemon over the salad and add the olive oil. Season with salt and pepper.

Nutrition Facts: Calories: 84 Carbs: 3g Fat: 4g Protein: 0g

Broccoli Salad

Preparation Time: 20 minutes

Cooking Time: 5 minutes

Servings: 1

Ingredients:

1 head of Broccoli

1/2 medium Red onion

2 Carrots, grated

¼ cup Red grapes

| 2 1/2 tbsp. Coconut yogurt | 1 tsp Mustard |
| 1 tbsp. Water | 1 pinch Salt |

Directions:

Cut the broccoli into small florets and cook for 8 minutes. Cut the red onion into thin half rings. Halve the grapes. Mix coconut yogurt, water and mustard with a pinch of salt to make the dressing.

Drain the broccoli and rinse with ice-cold water to stop the cooking process.

Mix the broccoli with the carrot, onion and red grapes in a bowl. Serve the dressing separately on the side.

Nutrition Facts: Calories: 230 Fat: 18g Carbohydrate: 35g Protein: 10g

Fresh Chicory Salad

Preparation Time: 10 minutes

Cooking Time: 0 minutes

Servings: 1

Ingredients:

½ medium red chicory	1/2 medium Cucumber
1 medium Orange	1/2 medium Red onion
1 large Tomato	

Directions:

Cut off the hard stem of the chicory and remove the leaves. Peel the orange and cut the pulp into wedges.

Cut the tomatoes and cucumbers into small pieces. Cut the red onion into thin half rings.

Place the chicory boats on a plate; spread the orange wedges, tomato, cucumber and red onion over the boats. Drizzle some olive oil and fresh lemon juice and serve.

Nutrition Facts: Calories: 112 Fat: 11g Carbohydrate: 2g Protein: 0g

Steak Salad

Preparation Time: 90 minutes

Cooking Time: 30 minutes

Servings: 4

Ingredients:

2 4 oz. Beef steak	2 tbsp. olive oil
2 cloves Garlic	1-ripe Avocado
1-medium Red onion	1/2 Cucumber
2 Eggs	1 pinch Salt and pepper
1 cup Cherry tomatoes	1 tbsp. white vinegar

Directions:

Place the steaks in a flat bowl. Pour the olive oil over the steaks and crush the garlic over. Turn the steaks a few times so that they are covered with oil and garlic. Cover the meat and let it marinate for at least 1 hour. Boil eggs until done, rinse and let cool.

Heat a grill pan and fry the steaks. When done, let them rest 5 minutes wrapped in aluminum foil. Spread the lettuce on the plates. Cut the steaks into slices and place them in the middle of the salad.

Cut the eggs into wedges, the cucumber into half-moons, the red onion into thin half-rings, the cherry tomatoes into halves and the avocado into slices.

Spread this around the steaks. Drizzle over the olive oil and white wine vinegar and season with a little salt and pepper.

Nutrition Facts: Calories: 513 Fat: 15g Carbohydrate: 1g Protein: 47g

Zucchini Salad With Lemon Chicken

Preparation Time: 90 minutes

Cooking Time: 30 minutes

Servings: 1

Ingredients:

2 zucchini, sliced

4 oz. Cherry tomatoes

5 oz. Chicken breast

1 Lemon

2 tbsp. Olive oil

1 tbsp. rosemary

1 clove of garlic, crushed

Salt and pepper to taste

Direction:

Use a meat mallet or a heavy pan to make the chicken fillets as thin as possible. Put the fillets in a bowl. Squeeze the lemon over the chicken and add the olive oil, salt, pepper, rosemary and garlic.

Cover it and let it marinate for at least 1 hour. Heat a pan over medium-high heat and fry the chicken until cooked through and browned.

Quarter the tomatoes and slice the zucchini and put everything in a serving plate. Slice the chicken fillets diagonally and place them on the salad.

Drizzle the salad with a little olive oil and season with salt and pepper.

Nutrition Facts: Calories: 286kcal Fat: 8g Carbohydrate: 4g Protein: 0g

Tuna Salad and Red Chicory

Preparation Time: 20 minutes

Cooking Time: 0 minutes

Servings: 2

Ingredients:

4 pieces Red chicory

5 oz. Tuna

1-piece Orange

1 tbsp. fresh parsley, finely chopped

5 pieces Radish

1 tsp Olive oil

Directions:

Drain the tuna. Cut the orange into wedges and and then into small pieces.

Cut radishes into small pieces too.

Mix all the ingredients (except the red chicory) in a small bowl. Season with salt and pepper

Spread the tuna mix on the red chicory leaves and enjoy!

Nutrition Facts: Calories: 93 Fat: 6g Carbohydrate: 2g Protein: 9g

Salad With Bacon, Cranberries And Apple

Preparation Time: 40 minutes

Cooking Time: 10 minutes

Servings: 3

Ingredients:

½ cup Arugula

4 slices Bacon

1/2 pieces Apple

2 tbsp. Dried cranberries

1/2 pieces Red onion

1/2 pieces Red bell pepper

10 Walnuts

Ingredients dressing:

1 tsp Mustard yellow

1 tsp Honey

3 tbsp. Olive oil

Directions:

Heat a pan over medium heat and fry the bacon until crispy. Place the bacon on a piece of kitchen roll so that the excess fat is absorbed. Cut half the red onion into thin rings. Cut the bell pepper into small cubes. Cut the apple into four pieces and remove the core. Then cut into thin wedges. Drizzle some lemon juice on the apple wedges so that they do not change color.

Roughly chop walnuts. Mix the ingredients for the dressing in a bowl. Season with salt and pepper. Spread the lettuce on a plate and season with red pepper, red onions, apple wedges and walnuts.

Sprinkle bacon and cranberries over the salad. Drizzle the dressing over the salad and serve.

Nutrition Facts: Calories: 70 Fat: 3g Carbohydrate: 6g Protein: 7g

Hawaii Salad

Preparation Time: 25 minutes

Cooking Time: 0 minutes

Servings: 1

Ingredients:

½ cup rocket

1/2 pieces Red onion

1-piece winter carrot

1 cup Pineapple

3 oz. ham, diced

1 pinch Salt

1 pinch Black pepper

Directions:

Cut the red onion into thin half rings. Remove the peel and hard core from the pineapple and cut the pulp into thin pieces. Clean the carrot and use a spiralizer to make strings.

Mix rocket and carrot in a bowl. Spread this over a plate. Spread red onion, pineapple and diced ham over the rocket.

Drizzle the olive oil and balsamic vinegar on the salad to your taste.

Season with salt and pepper.

Nutrition Facts: Calories: 200kcal Fat: 6g Carbohydrate: 28g Protein: 8g

Rainbow Salad

Preparation Time: 10 minutes

Cooking Time: 0 minutes

Servings: 1

Ingredients:

1 cup lettuce

1/2 pieces Avocado

1 Egg

1/4 pieces green peppers

1/4 pieces Red bell pepper

2 large Tomato

1/2 pieces Red onion

4 tbsp. Carrot, grated

2 tbsp olive oil

1 tbsp white vinegar

Salt

Pepper

Directions:

Boil the egg until done (6 minutes for soft boiled, 8 minutes for hard boiled). Cool it under running water, peel it and cut into slices.

Remove the seeds from the peppers and cut them into thin strips. Cut the tomatoes into small cubes. Cut the red onion into thin half rings.

Cut the avocado into thin slices.

Place the salad on a plate and distribute all the vegetables in colorful rows.

Drizzle the vegetables with olive oil and white wine vinegar. Season with salt and pepper.

Nutrition Facts: Calories: 40kcal Fat: 1g Carbohydrate: 5g Protein: 2g

Mung Beans Snack Salad

Preparation Time: 10 minutes

Cooking Time: 0 minutes

Servings: 6

Ingredients:

2 cups tomatoes, chopped

2 cups cucumber, chopped

3 cups mixed greens

2 cups mung beans, sprouted

2 cups clover sprouts

For the dressing:

1 tbsp. cumin, ground

1 cup dill, chopped

4 tbsp. lemon juice

1 avocado, pitted and roughly chopped

1 cucumber, roughly chopped

Directions:

In a salad bowl, mix tomatoes with 2 cups cucumber, greens, clover and mung sprouts.

In your blender, mix cumin with dill, lemon juice, 1 cucumber and avocado, blend really well, add this to your salad, toss well and serve.

Nutrition Facts: Calories 120 kcal, Fat 3g, Carbohydrate 10g, Protein 6g

Sprouts And Apples Snack Salad

Preparation Time: 10 minutes

Cooking Time: 0 minutes

Servings: 4

Ingredients:

- 1 lb. Brussels sprouts, shredded
- 1 cup walnuts, chopped
- 1 apple, cored and cubed
- 1 red onion, chopped
- 3 tbsp. red vinegar
- 1 tbsp. mustard
- ½ cup olive oil
- 1 garlic clove, crushed
- Black pepper to the taste

Directions:

In a salad bowl, mix sprouts with apple, onion and walnuts.

In another bowl, mix vinegar with mustard, oil, garlic and pepper, whisk really well, add this to your salad, toss well and serve as a snack.

Nutrition Facts: Calories 120 kcal, Fat 2g, Carbohydrate 8g, Protein 6g

Moroccan Leeks Snack Salad

Preparation Time: 10 minutes

Cooking Time: 0 minutes

Servings: 4

Ingredients:

1 bunch radishes, sliced

3 cups leeks, chopped

1 and ½ cups olives, pitted and sliced

A pinch of turmeric powder

1 cup cilantro, chopped

Salt to taste

Black pepper to taste

2 tbsp. olive oil

Directions:

In a bowl, mix radishes with leeks, olives and cilantro. Add black pepper, oil and turmeric, toss to coat and serve.

Nutrition Facts: Calories 135kcal, Fat 1g, Carbohydrate18g, Protein 9g

Celery And Raisins Snack Salad

Preparation Time: 10 minutes

Cooking Time: 0 minutes

Servings: 4

Ingredients:

½ cup raisins

4 cups celery, sliced

¼ cup parsley, chopped

½ cup walnuts, chopped

Juice of ½ lemon

2 tbsp. olive oil

Salt and black pepper to taste

Directions:

In a salad bowl, mix celery with raisins, walnuts, parsley, lemon juice, oil and black pepper, toss, divide into small cups and serve as a snack.

Nutrition Facts: Calories 120 kcal, Fat 1g, Carbohydrate 6g, Protein 5g

Dijon Celery Salad

Preparation Time: 10 minutes

Cooking Time: 0 minutes

Servings: 4

Ingredients:

½ cup lemon juice

1/3 cup Dijon mustard

2/3 cup olive oil

Black pepper to taste

2 apples, cored, peeled and cubed

1 bunch celery roughly chopped

¾ cup walnuts, chopped

Directions:

In a salad bowl, mix celery and its leaves with apple pieces and walnuts.

Add black pepper, lemon juice, mustard and olive oil, whisk well, add to your salad, toss, divide into small cups and serve.

Nutrition Facts: Calories 125 kcal, Fat 2g, Carbohydrate 7g, Protein 7g

Soups

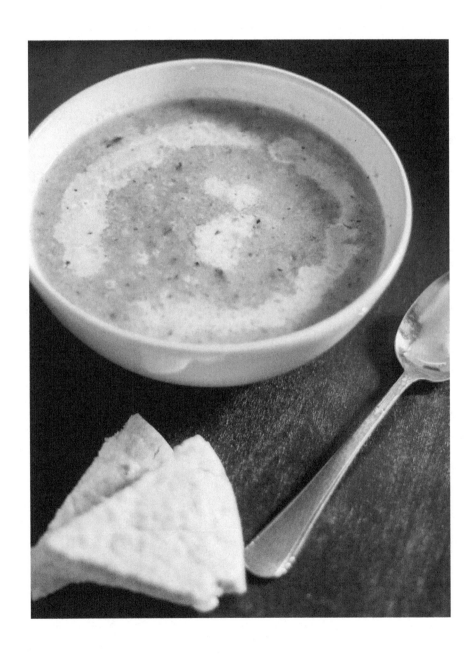

Kale, Apple And Fennel Soup

Preparation Time: 5 minutes

Cooking Time: 20 minutes

Servings: 4

Ingredients:

1 lb. kale, chopped

7 oz. fennel, chopped

2 apples, peeled, cored and chopped

2 tbsp. fresh parsley, chopped

1 tbsp. olive oil

Sea salt

Freshly ground black pepper

Directions:

Heat the oil in a saucepan, add the kale and fennel and cook for 5 minutes until the fennel has softened. Stir in the apples and parsley. Cover with hot water, bring it to the boil and simmer for 10 minutes.

Blitz in a food processor until the soup is smooth. Season with salt and pepper.

Nutrition Facts: Calories: 165kcal Fat: 9g Carbohydrate: 21g Protein: 3g

Lentil Soup

Preparation Time: 5 minutes

Cooking Time: 25 minutes

Servings: 4

Ingredients:

6 oz. red lentils

1 red onion, chopped

1 clove of garlic, chopped

2 sticks of celery, chopped

2 carrots, chopped

½ bird's eye chili

1 tsp. ground cumin

1 tsp. ground turmeric

1 tsp. ground coriander

2 pints vegetable stock

2 tbsp. olive oil

Salt and pepper

Directions:

Heat the oil in a saucepan and add the onion and cook for 5 minutes. Add in the carrots, lentils, celery, chili, coriander, cumin, turmeric and garlic and cook for 5 minutes.

Pour in the stock, bring it to the boil, reduce the heat and simmer for 45 minutes.

Blitz in a food processor until the soup is smooth

Season with salt and pepper and serve.

Nutrition Facts: Calories: 196kcal Fat: 4g Carbohydrates: 3g Protein: 3.4g

Cauliflower And Walnut Soup

Preparation Time: 5 minutes

Cooking Time: 15 minutes

Servings: 4

Ingredients:

1 lb. cauliflower, chopped

8 walnut halves, chopped

1 red onion, chopped

2 cups vegetable stock

3½ Fl. oz. double cream

½ tsp. turmeric

1 tbsp. olive oil

Directions:

Heat the oil in a saucepan, add the cauliflower and red onion and cook for 4 minutes, stirring continuously. Pour in the stock, bring to the boil and cook for 15 minutes. Stir in double cream and turmeric.

Using a food processor, blitz the soup until smooth and creamy.

Serve into bowls and top off with a sprinkling of chopped walnuts.

Nutrition Facts: Calories: 240kcal Fat: 5g Carbohydrate: 2g Protein: 3g

Celery And Blue Cheese Soup

Preparation Time: 5 minutes

Cooking Time: 25 minutes

Servings: 3

Ingredients:

4 oz blue cheese

1 oz butter

1 head of celery

1 red onion, chopped

1½ pints chicken stock

5fl oz. single cream

Directions:

Heat the butter in a saucepan, add the onion and celery and cook until the vegetables have softened.

Pour in the stock, bring to the boil then reduce the heat and simmer for 15 minutes.

Pour in cream and cheese and stir in the cheese until it has melted.

Serve and eat straight away.

Nutrition Facts: Calories: 340kcal Fat: 16g Carbohydrate: 41g Protein: 31g

Spicy Squash Soup

Preparation Time: 5 minutes

Cooking Time: 35 minutes

Servings: 4

Ingredients:

5oz kale

1 butternut squash, peeled, de-seeded and chopped

1 red onion, chopped

3 bird's eye chilies, chopped

3 cloves of garlic

2 tsp. turmeric

1 tsp. ground ginger

2 cups vegetable stock

2 tbsp. olive oil

Directions:

Heat the olive oil in a saucepan, add the chopped butternut squash and onion and cook for 6 minutes until softened.

Stir in the kale, garlic, chili, turmeric and ginger and cook for 2 minutes, stirring constantly.

Pour in the vegetable stock bring it to the boil and cook for 20 minutes. Using a food processor blitz the soup until smooth. Serve immediately.

Nutrition Facts: Calories: 298kcal Fat: 9g Carbohydrate: 24g Protein: 5g

French Onion Soup

Preparation Time: 5 minutes

Cooking Time: 25 minutes

Servings: 4

Ingredients:

2 lbs. red onions, thinly sliced

2 oz. cheddar cheese, grated

½ oz. butter

2 tsp. flour

2 slices whole wheat bread

1½ pints beef stock

1 tbsp. olive oil

Directions:

Heat the butter and oil in a large pan.

Add the onions and gently cook on low heat for 25 minutes, stirring occasionally. Add in the flour and stir well. Pour in the stock and keep stirring. Bring to the boil, reduce the heat and simmer for 30 minutes.

Cut the slices of bread into triangles, sprinkle with cheese and place them under a hot grill until the cheese has melted. Serve the soup into bowls and add 2 triangles of cheesy toast on top and enjoy.

Nutrition Facts: Calories: 210kcal Fat: 10g Carbohydrate: 18g Protein: 13g

Cream Of Broccoli & Kale Soup

Preparation Time: 5 minutes

Cooking Time: 35 minutes

Servings: 4

Ingredients:

9 oz. broccoli

9 oz. kale

1 potato, peeled and chopped

1 red onion, chopped

1 pint vegetable stock

½ pint milk

1 tbsp. olive oil

Sea salt

Freshly ground black pepper

Directions:

Heat the olive oil in a saucepan, add the onion and cook for 5 minutes. Add in the potato, kale and broccoli and cook for 5 minutes.

Pour in stock and milk and simmer for 20 minutes.

Using a food processor, blitz the soup until smooth and creamy. Season with salt and pepper. Serve immediately.

Nutrition Facts: Calories: 207kcal Fat: 12g Carbohydrate: 17g Protein: 9g

Chicken, Kale And Lentil Soup

Preparation Time: 5 minutes

Cooking Time: 25 minutes

Servings: 3

Ingredients:

5 cups vegetable stock

1 chicken breast, cooked and shredded

1 small red onion

2 cups of kale, finely chopped

1 cup of spinach, chopped

1 cup of lentils

1 celery stick, chopped

1 carrot, chopped

1 small chili pepper

A dash of salt

1 tsp. of extra virgin olive oil

Directions:

Boil the lentils according to the package but taking them out just a few minutes before they would be done. Set aside.

Add all the vegetables to a large pot, sauté in a bit of the oil on medium heat. Stir until the vegetables are softer but not cooked through.

Add the chicken and the lentils you had set aside, and cook for 3-5 minutes more.

Add a dash of the salt. Add the stock, turn down to low, and simmer for 20 minutes. Remove from heat. Serve when cooled.

Nutrition Facts: Calories: 199kcal Fat: 5g Carbohydrates: 20g Protein: 18g

Spicy Asian Noodle Soup

Preparation Time: 5 minutes

Cooking Time: 40 minutes

Servings: 2

Ingredients:

1 package buckwheat noodles, prepared as instructed on package

1 small red onion

2 stalks of celery, washed and chopped

1 chunk of ginger, diced

1 clove of garlic, minced

1 cup of arugula

¼ cup basil leaves, chopped

¼ cup of walnuts

1 tsp. of sesame seeds

2 tbsp. Blackcurrants

½ chili pepper

5 cups of chicken or vegetable stock

Juice of ½ lime

1 tsp. extra virgin olive oil

1 tbsp. of soy sauce

Directions:

Cook the noodles as instructed and set aside. In a pan, sauté all of the vegetables, ginger, garlic, chili, and nuts for about 10 minutes on very low heat.

Add the stock, and simmer for another 5 minutes.

Cut the noodles so that they are a size, small enough to eat in a soup comfortably. Add these to the soup, toss in the sesame seeds, lime juice and remove from heat. Serve warm.

Nutrition Facts: Calories: 220kcal Fat: 3g Carbohydrate: 23g Protein: 25g

Tofu And Shitake Mushroom Soup

Preparation Time: 5 minutes

Cooking Time: 30 minutes

Servings: 3

Ingredients:

½ oz. dried wakame seaweed

4 cups vegetable stock

8oz shiitake mushrooms, sliced

2 oz. miso paste

16oz firm tofu, diced

2 green onion, trimmed and diagonally chopped

1 bird's eye chili, finely chopped

Directions:

Soak the wakame in lukewarm water for 10-15 minutes before draining.

In a medium-sized saucepan add the vegetable stock and bring to the boil. Toss in the mushrooms and simmer for 2-3 minutes.

Mix the miso paste with 3-4 tbsp. of vegetable stock from the saucepan, until the miso is entirely dissolved.

Pour the miso-stock back into the pan and add the tofu, wakame, green onions and chili, then serve immediately.

Nutrition Facts: Calories: 203kcal Fat: 5g Carbohydrates: 32g Protein: 8g

Kale And Shiitake Soup

Preparation Time: 5 Minutes

Cooking Time: 40 minutes

Servings: 4

Ingredients:

1 cup kale

3 garlic cloves, minced

2 cups chopped onions

1/2 cup olive oil

Salt & 1 Tsp. ground pepper to taste

4 cups vegetable broth

2 pounds dry shiitake mushrooms

Directions:

Put oil, garlic, onion and kale in pan on medium heat, let them soften a few minutes.

Add mushrooms and sauté 2 minutes.

Add stock, bring to a boil and let simmer for 1 hour.

Serve immediately.

Nutrition Facts: Calories: 124kcal Fat: 2g Carbohydrate: 17g Protein: 9g

Turmeric Zucchini Soup

Preparation Time: 5 min

Cooking Time: 15 min

Servings: 2

Ingredients:

1 tbsp. extra virgin olive oil

½ tsp Sea salt

1 Large onion, diced

1 tbsp. Mild curry powder

3 cloves Garlic, diced

2 Medium zucchini, cubed

1 tbsp Fresh cilantro

¼ tsp White pepper

2 tsp Turmeric powder

2 tbsp. Lime juice

1 tsp Fish sauce

1 cup Coconut milk

1 cup Vegetable stock

Direction:

Place a saucepan over medium heat with olive oil. Once hot, add the onion and sauté for 5 minutes, occasionally stirring, until golden and soft.

Add the garlic, zucchini, and salt. Stir to mix with the onion.

Add pepper, curry powder, and turmeric and stir for some seconds to release the aromas. Now add the fish sauce, coconut milk, and vegetable stock and stir again.

Allow to boil, then reduce the heat to low. Cover with a lid and simmer for 10 minutes.

Add the lime juice and stir through. Garnish with a few fresh coriander leaves.

Nutrition Facts: Calories: 141kcal Fat: 11g Carbohydrates: 7g Protein: 4g

Kale And Stilton Soup

Preparation Time: 10 min

Cooking Time: 20 min

Servings: 4

Ingredients:

4oz Stilton Cheese, other cheese

1 large potato, chopped finely

2 cups kale, chopped

4 cups vegetable stock

3 tbsp. double cream

Fresh nutmeg

Direction:

Add the vegetable stock and the diced potatoes into a large pan cover with a lid and allow to boil, then cook for 10 minutes until the potato softens.

Add the crumbled stilton and chopped kale, cover, and cook for another five minutes.

Add the double cream, stir and add a generous amount of grounded fresh nutmeg—season to taste.

Use the back of your spoon to mash some of the potatoes.

Serve with some more crumbled stilton on top.

Nutrition Facts: Calories: 174kcal Fat: 8g Carbohydrate: 16g Protein: 7g

Tofu & Shiitake Mushroom Soup

Preparation Time: 30 minutes

Cooking Time: 3 minutes

Servings: 4

Ingredients:

⅜ oz. dried Wakame

32 fl. oz. vegetable stock

7 oz. shiitake mushrooms, sliced

4 ¼ oz. miso paste

14 oz. firm tofu, diced

2 green onion, chopped diagonally

1 bird's eye chili, finely chopped

Directions:

Soak the Wakame in lukewarm water for 15 minutes before draining.

In saucepan add the vegetable stock and bring to the boil. Toss in the mushrooms and simmer for 2-3 minutes.

Mix miso paste with 3-4 tbsp. of vegetable stock from the saucepan, until the miso is entirely dissolved.

Pour the miso-stock back into the pan and add the tofu, Wakame, green onions and chili, then serve immediately.

Nutrition Facts: Calories: 99 kcal Fat: 2.12 g Carbohydrates: 17.41 g Protein: 4.75 g

Snacks

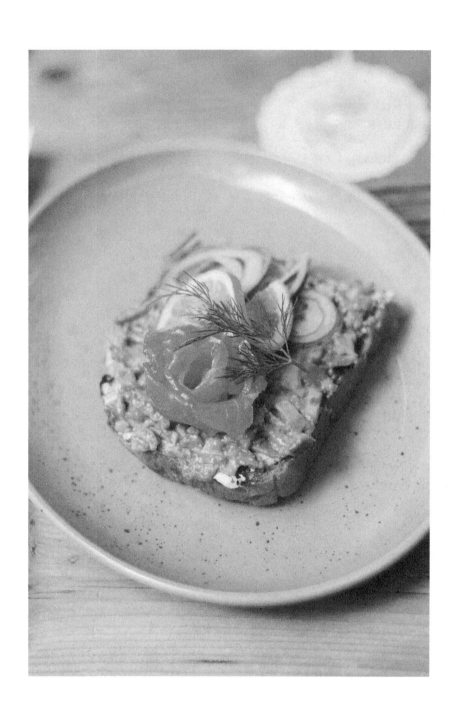

Sirtfood Granola

Preparation Time: 1 hour 10 minutes

Cooking Time: 50 minutes

Servings: 12

Ingredients:

7 oz. oats

9 oz. buckwheat flakes

3 ½ oz. walnuts, chopped

3 ½ oz. almonds, chopped

3 ½ oz. dried strawberries

1 ½ tsp. ground ginger

1 ½ tsp. ground cinnamon

4 fl. oz. extra virgin olive oil

2 tbsp. honey (optional)

Directions:

Preheat oven to 300°F. Line a tray with parchment paper. Stir together walnuts, almonds, buckwheat flakes and oats with ginger and cinnamon. In a large pan, warm olive oil and honey, heating until the honey has dissolved.

Pour the honey-oil over the other ingredients, stirring to ensuring an even coating. Distribute the granola evenly over the lined baking tray and roast for 50 minutes, or until golden.

Remove from the oven and leave to cool. Once cooled add the berries and store in an airtight container. Eat dry or with milk and yogurt. It stays fresh for up to 1 week.

Nutrition Facts: Calories: 178 kcal Fat: 10.9 g Carbohydrates: 22 g Protein: 6.7 g

Choc Chip Granola

Preparation Time: 45 minutes

Cooking Time: 30 minutes

Servings: 8

Ingredients

8oz jumbo oats

2oz pecans

3 tbsp. olive oil

1oz butter

1 tbsp. brown sugar

2 tbsp. rice malt syrup

2oz 70% chocolate chips

Directions

Preheat the oven to 325°.Line a large baking tray with parchment paper.

Mix the oats and pecans together in a huge bowl. In a small skillet, gently warm the olive oil, butter, brown sugar and rice malt butter till the butter has melted and the sugar and butter have simmer. Pour the syrup over the mix and stir thoroughly until the oats are fully covered.

Put the mix in baking tray and bake it in the oven for about 30 minutes until gold brown at the edges. Remove from the oven and leave to cool entirely.

Once cool, divide any larger lumps with your hands and mix in the chocolate chips. Put the granola in an airtight jar or tub. It will last around two weeks.

Nutrition Facts: Calories **220kcal** Fat 8g Carbohydrates 35g Protein 6g

Rosemary & Garlic Kale Chips

Preparation Time: 10 minutes

Cooking Time: 15 minutes

Servings: 6

Ingredients:

9oz kale chips, chopped

2 sprigs of rosemary

2 cloves of garlic

2 tbsp. olive oil

Sea salt

Freshly ground black pepper

Directions:

Gently warm the olive oil, rosemary and garlic over a low heat for 10 minutes. Remove it from the heat and set aside to cool.

Take the rosemary and garlic out of the oil and discard them.

Toss the kale leaves in the oil making sure they are well coated. Season with salt and pepper. Spread the kale leaves onto 2 baking sheets and bake them in the oven at 325F for 10 minutes, until crispy.

Nutrition Facts: Calories: 187kcal Fat: 13g Carbohydrates: 14g Protein: 6g

Honey Chili Nuts

Preparation Time: 25 minutes

Cooking Time: 10 minutes

Servings: 20

Ingredients:

5oz walnuts

5oz pecan nuts

2oz butter, softened

1 tbsp. honey

½ bird's-eye chili, very finely chopped

Directions:

Preheat the oven to 360F. Combine butter, honey and chili in a bowl then add the nuts and stir them well.

Spread the nuts onto a lined baking sheet and roast them in the oven for 10 minutes, stirring once halfway through. Remove from the oven and allow them to cool before eating.

Nutrition Facts: Calories: 260kcal Fat: 15g Carbohydrates: 20g Protein: 6g

Crunchy And Chewy Granola

Preparation Time: 45 minutes

Cooking Time: 60 minutes

Servings: 20

Ingredients:

1 tbsp. flax seeds

1/4 tsp. salt

1/2 tsp. cinnamon

1/2 cup honey

2 tbsp. brown-sugar

3/4 cup rolled oats

1/2 cup almonds, slivered

1/2 cup golden raisins

1/2 cup dried cranberries

Directions:

Pre-heat oven to 300°F. Line baking tray with parchment paper.

Mix flax seeds, cinnamon, honey, sugar oats and almonds. Insert 1 cup hot water, then mix together with hands. Spread into a thin layer over the baking tray.

Bake for 50-60 minutes, until gold brown. Remove from the oven and let cool.

Stir in dried fruit. Put the granola in an airtight jar or tub. It will last around two weeks.

Nutrition Facts: Calories: 233 Fat: 13g Carbohydrates: 31g Protein: 5g

Power Balls

Preparation Time: 15 minutes

Cooking Time: 2 minutes

Servings: 20

Ingredients:

1 cup old fashion oats

1/4 cup quinoa cooked using 3/4 cup orange juice

1/4 cup shredded unsweetened coconut

1/3 cup dried cranberry/raisin blend

1/3 cup dark chocolate chips

1/4 cup slivered almonds

1 tbsp. peanut butter

Directions:

Cook quinoa in orange juice. Bring to boil and simmer for approximately 15 minutes. Let cool. Combine quinoa and the remaining ingredients into a bowl.

With wet hands and combine ingredients and roll in ball sized chunks. Put in a container and let cool in the fridge for at least 2 hours before eating them.

Nutrition Facts: Calories: 189 Fat: 11g Carbohydrates: 22g Protein: 5g

Sirt Muesli

Preparation Time: 15 minutes

Cooking Time: 0 minutes

Servings: 1

Ingredients:

½ oz. buckwheat flakes

½ oz. buckwheat puffs

½ oz. shredded coconut

2 Medjool dates, pitted and chopped

4 walnuts, chopped

1tbsp cocoa nibs

4 oz. strawberries, hulled and chopped

4 oz. plain Greek yogurt

Directions:

Simply mix the dry ingredients and place them in an airtight container so that they are ready to eat. If you want, you can make it in bulk by multiplying the quantities.

To enjoy the sirt muesli, put the yogurt in bowl, put strawberries on top and then add the muesli.

Nutrition Facts: Calories: 368 Fat: 16g Carbohydrates: 54g Protein: 26g

Sirtfood Bites

Preparation Time: 35 minutes

Cooking Time: 0 minutes

Servings: 12

Ingredients:

4 oz. walnuts

1 oz. 85% dark chocolate

8 oz. Medjool dates, pitted

1 tbsp. cocoa powder

1 tbsp. ground turmeric

1 tbsp. extra virgin olive oil

1 tsp. vanilla extract, unsweetened

2 tbsp. water

Directions:

Put the walnuts and chocolate in a food processor and process until you have an even mixture.

Add all the remaining ingredients except water and combine until the mixture forms a disc.

Depending on the consistency of the mixture, you may or may not have to add the water; you don't want it to be too sticky.

Shape the mixture into bite-sized balls using your wet hands and roll them in cocoa powder.

Refrigerate for at least 1 hour in an airtight container before eating them.

They last up to 1 week in the fridge.

Nutrition Facts: Calories: 127kcal Fat: 6g Carbohydrates: 14g Protein: 4g

Dark Chocolate Pretzel Cookies

Preparation Time: 40 minutes

Cooking Time: 17 minutes

Servings: 4

Ingredients:

1 cup yogurt

1/2 tsp. baking soda

1/4 tsp salt

1/4 tsp. cinnamon

4 Tbsp. butter, softened

1/3 cup brown sugar

1 egg

1/2 tsp. vanilla

1/2 cup dark chocolate chips

1/2 cup pretzels chopped

Directions:

Pre Heat oven to 350°F.In a bowl, whisk together sugar, butter, vanilla, and egg. In another bowl, stir together the flour, baking soda, and salt.

Pour the liquid mix over the flour mix along with the chocolate chips and pretzels and stir until just blended.

Drop large spoonfuls of dough on a baking tray lined with parchment paper.

Bake for 15-17 minutes, or until the bottoms are crispy. Allow cooling on a wire rack.

Nutrition Facts: Calories: 290 Fat: 15g Carbohydrates: 36g Protein: 3g

Pear, Cranberry And Chocolate Crisp

Preparation Time: 40 minutes

Cooking Time: 45 minutes

Servings: 8

Ingredients:

1/2 cup flour

1/2 cup brown sugar

1 tsp. cinnamon

⅛ tsp. salt

3/4 cup yogurt

1/4 cup apples

1/3 cup butter, melted

1 tsp vanilla

1 tbsp. brown sugar

1/4 cup dried cranberries

1 tsp lemon juice

1 pear, diced

2 handfuls of dark chocolate chips

Directions:

Pre-heat oven to 375°F. Spray a casserole dish with a cooking spray. Put flour, sugar, cinnamon, salt, apple, yogurt and butter into a bowl and mix. Pour it on a baking tray lined with parchment paper.

In a large bowl, combine sugar, lemon juice, vanilla, pear, and cranberries. Pour this fruit mix along with chocolate chips over the baking tray. Bake for 45 minutes. until golden. Cool before serving.

Nutrition Facts: Calories: 239kcal Fat: 5g Carbohydrates: 46g Protein: 3g

Potato Bites

Preparation Time: 10 minutes

Cooking Time: 20 minutes

Servings: 3

Ingredients:

1 potato, sliced

2 bacon slices, cooked and crumbled

1 small avocado, pitted and cubed

Cooking spray

Directions:

Spread potato slices on a lined baking sheet, spray with cooking oil, introduce in the oven at 350°F, bake for 20 minutes, arrange on a platter, top each slice with avocado, and crumbled bacon and serve as a snack.

Nutrition Facts: Calories 180 kcal, Fat 4g, Carbohydrates 8g, Protein 6g

Dill Bell Pepper Snack Bowls

Preparation Time: 10 minutes

Cooking Time: 0 minutes

Servings: 4

Ingredients:

2 tbsp. dill, chopped

1 yellow onion, chopped

1 lb. bell peppers, cut into thin strips

3 tbsp. olive oil

2 and ½ tbsp. white vinegar

Black pepper to the taste

Directions:

In a salad bowl, mix bell peppers with onion, dill, pepper, oil, and vinegar, toss to coat, divide into small bowls and serve as a snack.

Nutrition Facts: calories 120 kcal, fat 3g, fiber 4g, carbs 2g, Protein 3g

Cocoa Bars

Preparation Time: 10min + 12 hours

Cooking Time: 0 minutes

Servings: 12

Ingredients:

1 cup unsweetened cocoa chips

2 cups rolled oats

1 cup low-fat peanut butter

½ cup chia seeds

½ cup raisins

¼ cup of coconut sugar

½ cup of coconut milk

Directions:

Put 1 cup oats in the blender, pulse and transfer to a bow.

Add the rest of the oats, cocoa chips, chia seeds, raisins, sugar and milk, stir well, spread into a square pan, press well, keep in the fridge for 12 hours, slice into 12 bars and serve.

Bars can also be put in the freezer.

Nutrition Facts: Calories 198 kcal Fat 5g, Carbohydrates 10g, Protein 89g

Cinnamon Apple Chips

Preparation Time: 10 minutes

Cooking Time: 2 hours

Servings: 4

Ingredients:

Cooking spray

2 teaspoons cinnamon powder

2 apples, cored and thinly sliced

Directions:

Arrange apple slices on a lined baking sheet, spray them with cooking oil, sprinkle cinnamon, introduce in the oven and bake at 300°F for 2 hours. Divide into bowls and serve as a snack.

Nutrition Facts: Calories 80kcal, Fat 0.5g, Carbohydrates 7g, Protein 4g

Cinnamon-Scented Quinoa

Preparation Time: 5 minutes

Cooking Time: 0 minutes

Servings: 4

Ingredients:

Chopped walnuts

1 ½ cup water

Maple syrup

2 cinnamon sticks

1 cup quinoa

Directions:

Add the quinoa to a bowl and wash it until the water is clear. Use a fine-mesh sieve to drain it.

Prepare your pressure cooker with a trivet and steaming basket. Place the quinoa and the cinnamon sticks in the basket and pour the water.

Close and lock the lid. Cook at high pressure for 6 minutes. When the cooking time is up, release the pressure using the quick release method.

Fluff the quinoa with a fork and remove the cinnamon sticks. Divide the cooked quinoa among serving bowls and top with maple syrup and chopped walnuts.

Nutrition Facts: Calories: 160, Fat: 3 g, Carbohydrates: 28 g, Protein: 6 g

No-Bake Choco Cashew Cheesecake

Preparation Time: 25 minutes

Cooking Time: 0 minutes

Servings: 8

Ingredients

2 cups raw cashews

¼ cup coconut cream

¼ cup unsweetened cocoa powder

¼ cup pure maple syrup

1 tsp vanilla extract

1¼ cups walnuts

¼ cup chopped dates

¼ tsp ground cinnamon

¼ cup almond meal

Directions:

Line the bottom of four 4-inch spring-form pans with a parchment paper circle.

Place cashews, coconut cream, cocoa powder, maple syrup and vanilla in a high-speed food processor. Repeat the process until it is entirely smooth, occasionally scraping the pieces with a rubber spatula. Transfer the mixture to a medium bowl and set aside. Clean the food processor or blender with a paper towel. This is the cream.

Place walnuts, dates, and cinnamon in the same food processor and blend quickly. This is the base.

Put the base mix in a baking tin. Create an even layer by pressing well. Pour in the cream and put in the fridge for 12 hours before enjoying it.

Nutrition Facts: Calories: 168kcal Fat: 11g Carbohydrates: 11g Protein: 7g

Cacao-Coated Almonds

Preparation Time: 10 minutes

Cooking Time: 15 minutes

Servings: 10

Ingredients:

¼ cup cocoa nibs

¼ cup light brown sugar

1 tsp instant espresso powder

Pinch of salt

2 teaspoons cornstarch

2 teaspoons warm water

1 tbsp. pure maple syrup

1 tsp pure vanilla extract, unsweetened

2 cups roasted whole almonds

Direction:

Preheat the oven to 325°F. Line a large baking tray with parchment paper.

Place the cocoa nibs, sugar, espresso powder, and salt in a coffee grinder. Grind to turn into a fine powder.

In a large bowl, whisk the cornstarch with the warm water until thoroughly combined. Stir the maple syrup and vanilla into the mixture. Add the almonds on top and fold until thoroughly coated.

Add the ground cacao mixture and combine until the almonds are thoroughly coated.

Place the almonds evenly on the baking tray. Toast for 10 minutes remove from the oven and stir gently. Toast for another 5 minutes or until the coating looks mostly dry. Be careful not to burn them! Let cool on the sheet. The coating will further harden once cooled. Store in an airtight container in the refrigerator for up to 2 weeks.

Nutrition Facts: Calories 132kcal, Fat 1g, Carbohydrate 6g, Protein 5g

Seed Crackers

Preparation Time: 30 minutes

Cooking Time: 8 minutes

Servings: 20

Ingredients

3 tbsp. white chia seeds

⅓ cup water

⅓ cup amaranth, cooked

⅓ cup whole wheat flour,

3 tbsp. shelled hemp seeds

3 tbsp. golden roasted flaxseeds

2 tbsp. almond flour

1½ teaspoons nutritional yeast

⅓ tsp fine sea salt

2 tbsp. olive oil

Direction:

Combine the chia seeds with the water in a small bowl. Let stand 2 minutes to thicken.

Add flour, amaranth, hemp seeds, flaxseed, almond flour, yeast, and salt. Add the thick mixture of chia and oil on top. Use a stand mixer with flat blades to mix perfectly and form a very sticky dough.

Wrap it tightly in a plastic wrap and refrigerate for 2 hours or (better) overnight.

Heat the oven to 400°F. Line two large baking trays with parchment paper. Divide the dough into 4 parts. Roll out a quarter super thin (0.5 inch) directly onto the baking tray. Use a cutter to cut the dough in rectangles.

Put the tray in the oven and cook for 8 minutes Repeat until you cooked all the dough. Allow cooling on a rack before stacking in an airtight container at room temperature. They will last for 5 days.

Nutrition Facts: Calories: 150kcal Fat: 8g Carbohydrates: 15g Protein: 4g

Spelt And Seed Rolls

Preparation Time: 20 minutes

Cooking Time: 2.5 hours +30 minutes

Servings: 9

Ingredients

1 cup almond milk, unsweetened,

2 tsp apple cider vinegar

⅓ cup water, lukewarm

2 tbsp. neutral-flavored oil

2 tbsp. agave nectar

⅓ cup whole spelt flour

¼ cup oat flour or finely ground oats

¼ cup vital wheat gluten

3 tbsp. shelled hemp seeds

3 tbsp. sunflower seeds

2 tbsp. golden roasted flaxseeds

2 tbsp. chia seeds

1 tbsp. poppy seeds

1 tsp fine sea salt

2 tsp instant yeast

Directions:

Combine milk and vinegar in a measuring cup. Allow 5 minutes to curdle. Filter curd, add water, oil and agave and set aside. In a bowl, place a flours, wheat gluten, seeds, salt, and yeast.

Mix them and the pour the wet mixture made with curd over.

Knead the dough with a stand mixer for 10 minutes until the dough becomes soft and not too dry or too sticky. If necessary, gently add 1 tbsp. of water until you get the desired result.

Cover and let it rest for 2 hours until doubled.

Divide the dough in 9 parts and give them the form of a roll and put them on a tray to rest for 25 minutes.

While the rolls rise, heat the oven to 400°F . When hot, cook the rolls for 20-22 minutes.

Let cool on a rack.

Store the rest in an airtight container at room temperature. They are best enjoyed fresh, but they will last up to 2 days.

Nutrition Facts: Calories: 140kcal Fat: 6g Carbohydrates: 14g Protein: 10g

Desserts

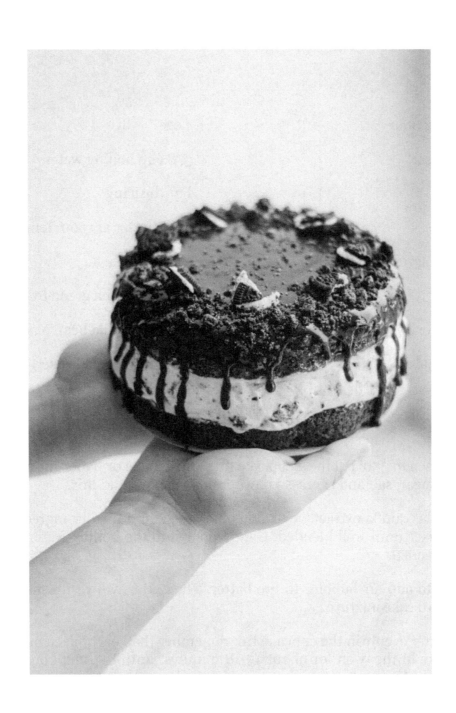

Chocolate Cupcakes With Matcha Icing

Preparation Time: 15 minutes

Cooking Time: 20 minutes

Servings: 12

Ingredients:

5 oz. self-rising flour

5 oz. caster sugar

2 oz. 60g cocoa

1/2 tsp salt

1/2 tsp. good espresso coffee

½ cup milk

½ tsp. vanilla extract, unsweetened

¼ cup vegetable oil

1 egg

3/8 cup boiling water

For the icing:

2 oz. butter at room temperature

2 oz. icing sugar

1 tbsp. matcha green tea powder

1/2 tsp. vanilla bean paste

50g soft cream cheese

Directions:

Preheat the oven to 350°F. Line a cupcake tin with silicone or paper muffin cups. Put the flour, cocoa, sugar, salt and espresso powder in a big bowl and mix.

Add the vanilla, vanilla extract, vegetable oil and egg into the dry ingredients beat with an electric mixer until well blended. Gently pour into the boiling water gradually until completely blended.

Keep mixing to add air bubbles to the batter. The batter will result much more liquid than a standard cake mixture.

Spoon the batter evenly in the cupcake tin, remember than each place must not be fuller than 3/4. Bake in the oven for about 15-18 minutes, until the mix bounces back when exploited.

Remove from the oven and let it cool completely before icing.

To make the icing, cream the butter and icing sugar together until smooth and soft. Add matcha powder vanilla and stir. Ice the cupcakes.

Nutrition Facts: Calories: 220kcal Fat: 8g Carbohydrate: 33g Protein: 4g

Fruit Skewers & Strawberry Dip

Preparation Time: 15 minutes

Cooking Time: 0 minutes

Servings: 6

Ingredients:

5oz red grapes

14oz strawberries

2lb pineapple, peeled and diced

Directions:

Place 3½ oz. of the strawberries into a food processor and blend until smooth. Pour the dip into a serving bowl. Skewer the grapes, pineapple chunks and remaining strawberries onto skewers. Serve alongside the strawberry dip.

Nutrition Facts: Calories: 131kcal Fat: 1g Carbohydrate: 30g Protein: 2g

Choc Nut Truffles

Preparation Time: 15 minute + 3 hours

Cooking Time: 0 minutes

Servings: 8

Ingredients:

5oz desiccated (shredded) coconut

2oz walnuts, chopped

1oz hazelnuts, chopped

4 medjool dates

2 tbsp. 100% cocoa powder or cacao nibs

1 tbsp. coconut oil

Directions:

Place all of the ingredients into a blender and process until smooth and creamy. Using a teaspoon, scoop the mixture into bite-size pieces then roll it into balls. Place them into small paper cups, cover them and chill for 3 hours before serving.

Nutrition Facts: Calories: 41kcal Fat: 3g Carbohydrate: 4g Protein: 1g

No-Bake Strawberry Flapjacks

Preparation Time: 15 minutes + 4 hours

Cooking Time: 0 minutes

Servings: 8

Ingredients:

3 oz. porridge oats

4 oz. dates

2 oz. strawberries

2 oz. peanuts, unsalted

2 oz. walnuts

1 tbsp. coconut oil

2 tbsp. 100% cocoa powder

Directions:

Place all of the ingredients into a blender and process until they become a soft consistency. Spread the mixture onto a baking sheet or small flat tin.

Press the mixture down and smooth it out. Put in the fridge 4 hours, then cut it into 8 pieces and serve.

Nutrition Facts: Calories: 191kcal Fat: 11g Carbohydrate: 21g Protein: 2g

Chocolate Balls

Preparation Time: 15 minutes

Cooking Time: 0 minutes

Servings: 6

Ingredients:

2oz peanut butter (or almond butter)

1oz cocoa powder

1oz desiccated (shredded) coconut

1 tbsp. honey

1 tbsp. cocoa powder for coating

Directions:

Place the ingredients into a bowl and mix. Using a tsp scoop out a little of the mixture and shape it into a ball. Roll the ball in a little cocoa powder and set aside. Repeat for the remaining mixture. Can be eaten straight away or stored in the fridge.

Nutrition Facts: Calories: 240 Carbs: 21g Fat: 15g Protein: 4g

Warm Berries & Cream

Preparation Time: 10 minutes

Cooking Time: 5 minutes

Servings: 4

Ingredients:

9oz blueberries

9oz strawberries

3½ oz. redcurrants

3½ oz. blackberries

4 tbsp. fresh whipped cream

1 tbsp. honey

Zest and juice of 1 orange

Directions:

Place all of the berries into a pan along with the honey and orange juice. Gently heat the berries for around 5 minutes until warmed through. Serve the berries into bowls and add a dollop of whipped cream on top.

Nutrition Facts: Calories: 217kcal Fat: 2g Carbohydrates: 30g Protein: 2g

Chocolate Fondue

Preparation Time: 5 minutes

Cooking Time: 5 minutes

Servings: 4

Ingredients:

4oz dark chocolate

11oz strawberries

7oz cherries

2 apples, peeled, cored and sliced

3½ Fl. oz. double cream

Directions:

Place the chocolate and cream into a saucepan and warm it until smooth and creamy. Serve in the fondue pot or transfer it to a serving bowl. Scatter the fruit on a serving plate ready to be dipped into the chocolate.

Nutrition Facts: Calories: 350kcal Fat: 10g Carbohydrates: 23g Protein: 2g

Walnut & Date Loaf

Preparation Time: 30 minutes

Cooking Time: 45 minutes

Servings: 12

Ingredients:

9oz self-rising flour

4oz medjool dates, chopped

2oz walnuts, chopped

8fl oz. milk

3 eggs

1 medium banana, mashed

1 tsp baking soda

Directions:

Sieve baking soda and flour into a bowl. Add in banana, eggs, milk and dates and mix well. Transfer the mixture to a lined loaf tin and smooth it out. Scatter the walnuts on top. Bake the loaf in the oven at 180C/360F for 45 minutes.

Transfer it to a wire rack to cool before serving.

Nutrition Facts: Calories: 186kcal Fat: 5g Carbs: 33g Protein: 2g

Strawberry Frozen Yogurt

Preparation Time: 60 – 120 minutes

Cooking Time: 0 minutes

Servings: 4

Ingredients:

1lb plain yogurt

6oz strawberries

Juice of 1 orange

1 tbsp. honey (optional)

Directions:

Place strawberries and orange juice into a food processor and blitz until smooth.

Filter the mixture through a sieve into a bowl to remove seeds. Stir in the honey and yogurt.

Transfer the mixture to an ice-cream maker and follow the manufacturer's instructions. Alternatively pour the mixture into a container and place in the freezer for 1 hour.

Use a fork to whisk it and break up ice crystals and freeze for other 2 hours.

Nutrition Facts: Calories: 100kcal Fat: 0.6g Carbohydrate: 21g Protein: 4g

Chocolate Brownies

Preparation Time: 15 minutes

Cooking Time: 30 minutes

Servings: 14

Ingredients

7oz dark chocolate (min 85% cocoa)

7oz medjool dates, pitted

3½oz walnuts, chopped

3 eggs

1fl oz. melted coconut oil

2 teaspoons vanilla essence

½ tsp baking soda

Directions:

Place the dates, chocolate, eggs, coconut oil, baking soda and vanilla essence into a food processor and mix until smooth.

Stir the walnuts into the mixture. Pour the mixture into a lined baking tray and bake at 350F for 25-30 minutes.

Allow it to cool. Cut into pieces and serve.

Nutrition Facts: Calories: 188kcal Fat: 12g Carbohydrate: 19g Protein: 3g

Crème Brûlée

Preparation Time: 10 minutes

Cooking Time: 3 minutes

Servings: 4

Ingredients:

14oz strawberries

11oz plain low-fat yogurt

4oz Greek yogurt

3½oz brown sugar

1 tsp vanilla extract

Directions:

Divide the strawberries between 4 ramekin dishes.

In a bowl combine the plain yogurt with the vanilla extract. Spoon the mixture onto the strawberries.

Scoop the Greek yogurt on top. Sprinkle the sugar over each dish, completely covering the top.

Place the dishes under a hot grill (broiler) for around 3 minutes or until the sugar has caramelized.

Nutrition Facts: Calories: 311kcal Fat: 25g Carbohydrate: 16g Protein: 5g

Pistachio Fudge

Preparation Time: 10 minutes

Cooking Time: 0 minutes

Servings: 6

Ingredients:

8oz medjool dates, pitted

3½ oz. pistachio nuts, shelled

2 oz. desiccated shredded coconut

1 oz. oats

2 tbsp. water

Directions:

Place the dates, nuts, coconut, oats and water into a food processor and process until the ingredients are well mixed.

Roll the mixture in a 1-inch thick roll a cut it into 6 pieces.

Refrigerate 2 hours and serve.

Nutrition Facts: Calories: 280kcal Fat: 12g Carbohydrate: 18g Protein: 4g.

Spiced Poached Apples

Preparation Time: 30 minutes

Cooking Time: 20 minutes

Servings: 4

Ingredients:

4 apples

2 tbsp. honey

4-star anise

2 cinnamon sticks

1 cup green tea

¼ cup Greek yogurt

Direction:

Place the honey and green tea into a saucepan and bring to the boil. Add apples, star anise and cinnamon. Reduce the heat and simmer gently for 15 minutes. Serve the apples with a dollop of Greek yogurt.

Nutrition Facts: Calories: 180 Fat: 0.5g Carbohydrate: 25g Protein: 5g

Banana Pecan Muffins

Preparation Time: 30 minutes

Cooking Time: 40 minutes

Servings: 8

Ingredients:

3 Tbsp. butter softened	2 cups flour
4 ripe bananas	1 tbsp. instant yeast
1 Tbsp. honey	2 pecans, sliced
⅛ cup orange juice, unsweetened	1 tbsp. vanilla
1 tsp cinnamon	2 eggs

Directions:

Preheat the oven to 350°F. Lightly oil sides and bottom of a muffin tin and dust with flour. Tap to remove any excess flour.

Peel the bananas and mash them with a in a bowl. Add flour and mix.

Add orange juice, butter, eggs, vanilla, yeast and cinnamon and stir to combine.

Roughly chop the pecans onto a chopping board, add to the mix.

Fill each muffin tin until 3/4 and bake in the oven for approximately 40 minutes, or until golden.

Nutrition Facts: Calories: 223kcal Fat: 9g Carbohydrates: 31g Protein: 7g

Banana And Blueberry Muffins

Preparation Time: 20 minutes

Cooking Time: 30 minutes

Servings: 12

Ingredients:

4 large ripe bananas, mashed

3/4 cup of sugar

1 egg, lightly beaten

1/2 cup of peanut butter,

2 cups of blueberries

1 tsp baking powder

1 tsp baking soda

1/2 tsp salt

1 cup of coconut, shredded

1/2 cup of flour

1/2 cup applesauce

Dab of cinnamon

Direction:

Add mashed banana to a large mixing bowl. Insert sugar and egg and mix well. Add peanut butter and blueberries.

Add the dry ingredients into the wet mix and mix together lightly.

Set into 12 greased muffin cups and bake for 20-25min at 350 F.

Nutrition Facts: Calories: 250 Carbs: 39g Fat: 9g Protein: 4g

Golden Milk Ice Cream

Preparation Time: 8 hours

Cooking Time: 5 min

Servings: 5

Ingredients:

28 oz. Full-fat coconut milk

2 tbsp. Extra virgin olive oil

1/4 cup Maple syrup

2-inchFresh ginger, finely sliced

A pinch of sea salt

½ tsp Ground cinnamon

1 tsp Ground turmeric

1/8 tsp Black pepper

1/8 tsp Cardamom

1 tsp pure vanilla extract, unsweetened

Directions:

Place your ice cream churn and bowl in the freezer a night before, to properly chill.

Add the maple syrup, turmeric, coconut milk, cardamom, fresh ginger, pepper, sea salt, and cinnamon into a large pot and heat over medium heat.

Allow to simmer, whisking continuously to mix the ingredients.

Then put off heat and add the vanilla extract. Stir once more to combine.

Adjust flavor if needed, adding more maple syrup for sweetness, turmeric for intense flavor, salt to balance the flavors, or cinnamon for warmth.

Transfer the mixture plus the ginger slices into a mixing bowl and allow to cool to room temperature.

Cover the bowl and place in the refrigerator to chill overnight or for a minimum of 4 to 6 hours.

The next day, use a strainer or a spoon to remove the ginger slices.

Then add the olive oil for more creaminess. Whisk to combine thoroughly.

Add the mixture to your ice cream maker and churn according to the instructions by the manufacturers – this should take about 30 minutes.

In case you don't have an ice cream maker, skip this phase and go to the next one.

Move the ice cream to a freezer-safe container and smoothen the top with your spoon.

Cover with a lid and place in the freezer for about four to six hours, until firm. Bring out of the freezer ten minutes before serving to soften.

Nutrition Facts: Calories: 140kcal Fat: 7g Carbohydrate: 17g Protein: 2g

Chocolate Cashew Truffles

Preparation Time: 10 minutes

Cooking Time: 35 minutes

Servings: 4

Ingredients:

1 cup ground cashews

1 tsp of ground vanilla bean

½ cup of coconut oil

¼ cup raw honey

2 flax meal

2 hemp hearts

2 cacao powder

Directions:

Mix all ingredients and make truffles by rolling small amounts of mixture and balls. Sprinkle coconut flakes on top.

Nutrition Facts: Calories: 187kcal Fat: 16.5g Carbohydrate: 6g Protein: 2.3g

Double Almond Raw Chocolate Tart

Preparation Time: 10 minutes

Cooking Time: 35 minutes

Servings: 4

Ingredients:

1½ cups of raw almonds

¼ cup of coconut oil, melted

1 raw honey

8 oz. dark chocolate, chopped

1 cup of coconut milk

½ cup unsweetened shredded coconut

Directions:

Crust:

Ground almonds and add melted coconut oil, raw honey and combine. Using a spatula spread this mixture into a pie pan.

Filling:

Put the chopped chocolate in a bowl, heat coconut milk and pour over chocolate and whisk together. Pour filling into tart shell. Refrigerate. Toast almond slivers chips and sprinkle over tart.

Nutrition Facts: Calories: 291 Fat: 9.4g Carbohydrate: 23.4g Protein: 12.4g

Bounty Bars

Preparation Time: 10 minutes

Cooking Time: 35 minutes

Servings: 4

Ingredients:

2 cups desiccated coconut

3 coconut oil - melted

1 cup of coconut cream - full fat

4 of raw honey

1 tsp ground vanilla bean

Coating:

Pinch of sea salt

½ cup cacao powder

2 raw honey

1/3 cup of coconut oil (melted)

Directions:

Mix coconut oil, coconut cream, and honey, vanilla and salt. Pour over desiccated coconut and mix well.

Mold coconut mixture into balls and freeze. Or pour the whole mixture into a tray, freeze and cut into small bars when frozen.

Prepare the coating by mixing salt, cocoa powder, honey and coconut oil. Dip frozen coconut balls/bars into the chocolate coating, put on a tray and freeze again.

Nutrition Facts: Calories: 120 Fat: 4.3g Carbohydrates: 16.7g Protein: 1g

Chocolate Cream

Preparation Time: 10 minutes

Cooking Time: 35 minutes

Servings: 4

Ingredients:

- 1 avocado
- 2 coconut oil
- 2 raw honey
- 2 cacao powder

- 1 tsp ground vanilla bean
- Pinch of salt
- ¼ cup almond milk
- ¼ cup goji berries

Directions:

Blend all the ingredients in the food processor until smooth and thick.

Distribute in four cups, decorate with goji berries and put the fridge overnight.

Nutrition Facts: Calories: 200kcal Fat: 4.3g Carbohydrate: 25.2g Protein: 12.8g

Peanut Butter Truffles

Preparation Time: 10 minutes

Cooking Time: 30 minutes

Servings: 4

Ingredients:

5 tbsp peanut butter

1 tbsp coconut oil

1 tbsp raw honey

1 tsp ground vanilla bean

¾ cup almond flour

Coating:

Pinch of salt

1 cocoa butter

½ cup 70% chocolate

Directions:

Mix peanut butter, c all ingredients in a dough.

Roll the dough into 1-inch balls, place them on parchment paper and refrigerate for half an hour (yield about 12 truffles).

Melted chocolate and cocoa butter, add a pinch of salt. Dip each truffle in the melted chocolate, one at the time. Place them back on the pan with parchment paper and put in the fridge.

Nutrition Facts: Calories: 194 Fat: 8g Carbohydrate: 13.1g Protein: 4g

Chocolate Pie

Preparation Time: 10 minutes

Cooking Time: 30 minutes

Servings: 4

Ingredients:

2 cups flour

1 cup dates, soaked and drained

1 cup dried apricots, chopped

1½ tsp ground vanilla bean

2 eggs

1 banana, mashed

5 cocoa powder

3 raw honey

1 ripe avocado, mashed

2 tbsp. organic coconut oil

½ cup almond milk

Directions:

In a bowl, add flour, apricots and dates finely chopped and mix. Add the banana and the eggs lightly beaten and mix.

Add vanilla, cocoa, honey, avocado and coconut oil and mix.

Add almond milk bit by bit. You could need less than ½ cup to get the right "cake consistency".

Put in a greased baking tin and cook for 30-35 minutes at 350° F. Always check the cake and allow a few more minutes if it's not done.

Allow to cool before serving.

Nutrition Facts: Calories: 380kcal Fat: 18.4g Carbohydrate: 50.2g Protein: 7.2g

Chocolate Walnut Truffles

Preparation Time: 10 minutes

Cooking Time: 35 minutes

Servings: 4

Ingredients:

1 cup ground walnuts

1 tsp cinnamon

½ cup of coconut oil

¼ cup raw honey

2 chia seeds

2 cacao powder

Directions:

Mix all ingredients and make truffles. Coat with cinnamon, coconut flakes or chopped almonds.

Nutrition Facts: Calories: 120kcal Fat: 4.4g Carbohydrate: 10.2g Protein: 5.2g

Frozen Raw Blackberry Cake

Preparation Time: 10 minutes

Cooking Time: 45 minutes

Servings: 4

Ingredients:

Crust:

3⁄4 cup shredded coconut

15 dried dates soaked and drained

1/3 cup pumpkin seeds

1⁄4 cup of coconut oil

Coconut whipped cream

Top filling:

1 pound of frozen blackberries

3⁄4 cup raw honey

1⁄4 cup of coconut cream

2 egg whites

Directions:

Grease the cake tin with coconut oil and mix all base ingredients in the blender until you get a sticky ball. Press the base mixture in a cake tin. Freeze. Make Coconut Whipped Cream. Freeze.

Blitz berries and then add honey, coconut cream and egg whites.

Pour middle filling - Coconut Whipped Cream in and spread evenly. Freeze. Pour top filling berries mixture-in the tin, spread, decorate with blueberries and almonds and return to freezer.

Nutrition Facts: Calories: 472 Fat: 18g Carbohydrate: 15.8g Protein: 33.3g

Chocolate Hazelnuts Truffles

Preparation Time: 10 minutes

Cooking Time: 30 minutes

Servings: 12

Ingredients:

1 cup ground almonds

1 tsp ground vanilla bean

½ cup of coconut oil

½ cup mashed pitted dates

12 whole hazelnuts

2 cacao powder

Directions:

Mix all ingredients and make truffles with one whole hazelnut in the middle.

Nutrition Facts: Calories: 70 Fat: 2.8g Net carbs: 16.9g Protein: 2.2g

Chocolate Pudding with Fruit

Preparation Time: 10 minutes

Cooking Time: 45 minutes

Servings: 2

Ingredients:

Chocolate cream:

1 avocado

2 tsp. raw honey

2 tbsp. coconut oil

3 tsp. cacao powder

1 tsp ground vanilla bean

Pinch of sea salt

¼ cup of coconut milk

Fruits:

1 chopped banana

1 cup pitted cherries

1 tbsp. coconut flakes

Directions:

Blend all chocolate cream ingredients and divide it in two cups.

Put fruit chunks on top and sprinkle shredded coconut on top.

Put at least 2 hours in the fridge before serving.

Nutrition Facts: Calories: 106kcal Fat: 5g Carbohydrate: 20.4g Protein: 14g

Chocolate Maple Walnuts

Preparation Time: 15 minutes

Cooking Time: 30 minutes

Servings: 15

Ingredients:

½ cup pure maple syrup,

2 cups raw, whole walnuts

½ cup dark chocolate, at least 85%

1 ½ tbsp. coconut oil, melted

1 tbsp. water

1 tsp. of vanilla extract

Directions:

Line a large baking sheet with parchment paper. In a medium to a large skillet, combine the walnuts and ¼ cup of maple syrup and cook over medium heat, stirring continuously, until walnuts are entirely covered with syrup and golden in color, about 3 – 5 minutes.

Pour the walnuts onto the parchment paper and separate it into individual pieces with a fork. Allow cooling completely; at least 15 minutes.

In the meantime, melt the chocolate with the coconut oil, add the remaining maple syrup and stir until combined. When walnuts are cooled, transfer them to a glass bowl and pour the melted chocolate syrup over the top.

Use a silicone spatula to mix until walnuts are entirely covered gently.

Transfer back to the parchment paper-lined baking sheet and, once again, separate each of the nuts with a fork.

Place the nuts in the fridge for 10 minutes or the freezer for 3 – 5 minutes, until chocolate has completely set. Store in an airtight bag in your fridge.

Nutrition Facts: Calories 139 Fat 10 g Carbohydrate 19 g Protein 24 g

Matcha and Chocolate Dipped Strawberries

Preparation Time: 25 minutes

Cooking Time: 25 minutes

Servings: 5

Ingredients:

4 tbsp. cocoa butter

4 squares of dark chocolate,

¼ cup of coconut oil

1 tsp Matcha green tea powder

20 – 25 large strawberries, stems on

Directions:

Melt cocoa butter, dark chocolate, coconut oil and Matcha until smooth. Remove from heat and continue stirring until chocolate is completely melted.

Pour into a large glass bowl and continuously stir until the chocolate thickens and starts to lose its sheen, about 2 - 5 minutes.

One at a time, hold the strawberries by stems and dip into chocolate matcha mixture to coat. Let excess drip back into the bowl.

Place on a parchment-lined baking sheet and chill dipped berries in the fridge until the shell is set, 20–25 minutes.

Nutrition Facts: Calories 188 Fat 5.3 g Carbohydrate 10.9 g Protein 0.2 g

Strawberry Rhubarb Crisp

Preparation Time: 10 minutes

Cooking Time: 45 minutes

Servings: 8

Ingredients:

1 cup white sugar

½ cup buckwheat flour + 3 tbsp.

3 cups strawberries, sliced

3 cups rhubarb, diced

½ lemon, juiced

1 cup packed brown sugar

1 cup coconut oil, melted

¾ cup rolled oats

¼ cup buckwheat groats

¼ cup walnuts, chopped

Directions:

Preheat oven to 375°F In a large bowl, mix white sugar, 3 tbsp. flour, strawberries, rhubarb, and lemon juice. Place the mixture in a 9x13 inch baking tray.

In a separate bowl, mix ½ cup flour, brown sugar, coconut oil, oats, buckwheat groats, and walnuts until crumbly.

Crumble on top of the rhubarb and strawberry mixture. Bake 45 minutes in the preheated oven, or until crisp and lightly browned.

Nutrition Facts: Calories 167 Fat 3.1 g Carbohydrate 58.3 g Protein 3.5 g

Maple Walnut Cupcakes with Matcha Green Tea Icing

Preparation Time: 20 minutes

Cooking Time: 25 minutes

Servings: 24

Ingredients:

For the Cupcakes:

2 cups of All-Purpose flour

½ cup buckwheat flour

2 ½ teaspoons baking powder

½ tsp salt

1 cup of cocoa butter

1 cup white sugar

1 tbsp. pure maple syrup

3 eggs

2/3 cup milk

¼ cup walnuts, chopped

For the Icing:

3 tbsp. coconut oil, thick at room temperature

3 tbsp. icing sugar

1 tbsp. Matcha green tea powder

½ tsp vanilla bean paste

3 tbsp. cream cheese, softened

Directions:

Preheat oven to 350 degrees F. Place paper baking cups into muffin tins for 24 regular-sized muffins. In a medium bowl, mix flours, baking powder, and salt.

In a separate large bowl, mix sugar, butter, syrup, and eggs with a mixer. Add to the dry ingredients, mix and add milk. Pour batter into muffin cup until 2/3 full.

Bake for 20-25 minutes or until an inserted toothpick comes out clean. Cool completely before icing. To Make the Icing: Add the coconut oil and icing sugar to a bowl and use a hand-mixer to cream until it's pale and smooth.

Fold in the matcha powder and vanilla. Finally, add the cream cheese and beat until smooth. Pipe or spread over the cupcakes once they're cool.

Nutrition Facts: Calories 164 Fat 6 g Carbohydrate 21 g Protein 2 g

Dark Chocolate Mousse

Preparation Time: 10 minutes

Cooking Time: 2+ hours

Servings: 4

Ingredients:

1 (16 oz.) package silken tofu, drained

½ cup pure maple syrup

1 tsp pure vanilla extract

¼ cup of soy milk

½ cup unsweetened cocoa powder

Mint leaves

Directions:

Place the tofu, maple syrup, and vanilla in a food processor or blender. Process until well blended.

Add remaining ingredients and process until the mixture is thoroughly blended.

Pour into small dessert cups or espresso cups. Chill for at least 2 hours. Garnish with fresh mint leaves just before serving.

Nutrition Facts: Calories 175kcal Fat 24 g Carbohydrate 18 g Protein 5 g

Matcha Green Tea Mochi

Preparation Time: 10 min

Cooking Time: 20 min

Servings: 12 pieces

Ingredients:

2 tbsp. Matcha powder.

1 cup superfine white rice flour

1 tsp Baking powder

1 cup Coconut milk

1/2 cup Sugar

2 tbsp. Butter melted

Directions:

Heat your oven to 325 degrees F. Grease your baking tin with a non-stick spray. Mix all the dry ingredients plus the sugar.

Whisk to blend, then add the coconut milk and melted butter. Stir well.

Place the mixture into the baking tin and place in the oven to bake for approx. 20 minutes.

Nutrition Facts: Calories: 100kcal Carbs: 13g Fat: 8g Protein: 2g

Appendix A - Conversion Tables

1. MEASUREMENT

Cups	Ounces	Milliliters	Tablespoons
8 cup	64 oz.	1895 ml	128 tbsp.
6 cup	48 oz.	1420 ml	96 tbsp.
5 cup	40 oz.	1180 ml	80 tbsp.
4 cup	32 oz.	960 ml	64 tbsp.
2 cup	16 oz.	480 ml	32 tbsp.
1 cup	8 oz.	240 ml	16 tbsp.
¾ cup	6 oz.	177 ml	12 tbsp.
2/3 cup	5 oz.	158 ml	11 tbsp.
½ cup	4 oz.	118 ml	8 tbsp.
3/8 cup	3 oz.	90 ml	6 tbsp.
1/3 cup	2.5 oz.	79 ml	5.5 tbsp.
¼ cup	2 oz.	59 ml	4 tbsp.
1/8 cup	1 oz.	30 ml	3 tbsp.
1/16 cup	½ oz.	15 ml	1 tbsp.